Couples in Conflict

In the first book of its kind, Dr. Stephen J. Betchen teaches established and training marriage and family therapists to recognize the complexity and contradictions of control struggles in couples and, uniquely, how to clinically treat these issues to create a harmonious, long relationship.

Integrating conflict theory, psychodynamic systems work, and the basic principles of sex therapy, the book aims to help professionals recognize and assess control struggles in couples, detect and examine their origin, and offer techniques to help break the struggle and alleviate its associated symptoms. Chapters begin by defining control and where the origin of control comes from before exploring how these origins and other sociocultural factors impact how we choose our partners. The book's second half examines how clinicians should assess and treat couples with both sexual and nonsexual symptoms, how to avoid being caught in the control crossfire as a therapist, and how to terminate sessions and prevent relapses.

Filled with case studies and useful interventions throughout, this book aims to help clinicians working with all couples across cultures and sexual orientations find a common ground. It is indispensable for training and graduate clinicians that work with couples, especially couples with sexual disorders.

Stephen J. Betchen, DSW, is a licensed marriage and family therapist, an AAMFT-approved supervisor, and an AASECT diplomate and certified supervisor. For many years he served as a senior supervisor in the post-graduate Sex Therapy Program at the Council for Relationships and as an adjunct clinical professor in the Department of Couple and Family Therapy at Thomas Jefferson University. He currently maintains a full-time private practice in New Jersey specializing in couples and sex therapy.

Couples in Conflict

Clinical Techniques for Navigating Sexual and Relationship Control Struggles

Stephen J. Betchen

Routledge
Taylor & Francis Group

NEW YORK AND LONDON

Cover image: Getty Images

First published 2022
by Routledge
605 Third Avenue, New York, NY 10158

and by Routledge
4 Park Square, Milton Park, Abingdon, Oxon, OX14 4RN

Routledge is an imprint of the Taylor & Francis Group, an informa business

Library of Congress Cataloging-in-Publication Data
A catalog record for this book has been requested

ISBN: 978-0-367-74338-3 (hbk)
ISBN: 978-0-367-74689-6 (pbk)
ISBN: 978-1-003-15910-0 (ebk)

DOI: 10.4324/9781003159100

Typeset in Times New Roman
by Apex CoVantage, LLC

To Walden Holl, Jr., M.D.

—Who taught me to try without guarantee, and to take the good with the bad.

Contents

Preface

In treating couples for a little over 40 years both in private practice and in various clinics, I have seen many of them "stuck" in a circular dynamic—like a two-person Ferris wheel that keeps on spinning. One partner attacks the other which in turn provokes a counterattack and vice versa. I refer to this dynamic as a process because a couple may demonstrate this interaction in a variety of contexts or by using different forms of content; in this book context and content are used interchangeably. For example, a couple can repeatedly joust about finances, politics, or sex. The process tends to stay the same, but the context or content may change. Some of these interactions become quite heated, and in their extreme, physical. Many of these couples have been in treatment with different clinicians, both behavioral and psychodynamic in orientation; others have added individual treatment to break their gridlock but were met with limited success. But what holds these couples in place? What is responsible for the symptoms that cause them to suffer?

In *Couples in Conflict*, I offer one perspective—a unique position that I hope will resonate with my professional colleagues. All couples are prone to battle over control from time to time. But I officially pronounce a "control struggle" when each partner is conflicted about control. That is, when one part of each person wants control, and the other part is uncomfortable having it, and as a collective unit the couple are unable to balance this conflict in a way that is comfortable. This imbalance must last long enough and be intense enough to produce relationship symptoms. I refer to this dominant, internal conflict as the couple's master conflict. I also believe that partners are attracted to and choose each other because they share this master conflict. I refer to them as twins-in-conflict.

Challenging a couple's unbalanced master conflict and breaking their chronic struggle for control is one of the most challenging dynamics in couples treatment; and I believe that my colleagues and supervisees would agree. The two primary reasons for this are: (1) because both partners collude in maintaining the conflict to avoid the pain that comes with change, which is perceived to be greater than the pain associated with their relationship symptoms; and (2) because the conflict is internalized, and for the most part, unconscious. For these reasons alone, couples can remain stuck in a control struggle for years only to frustrate themselves and any clinician who attempts to help them out of this paralyzing dynamic.

Nearly every book on couples therapy mentions the concept of control, but perplexing as it is, there has yet to be a professional book solely dedicated to the subject. *Couples in Conflict* fills that void by presenting an integrative (e.g., couples/sex therapy), systemic treatment model specifically designed to break a couple's battle for control, and to alleviate any associated symptoms. Unlike many books dedicated to couples therapy, if sexual symptoms present themselves, clinical interventions are offered including the incorporation of sex therapy exercises. My stance has always been that because couples often present with sexual difficulty, a couples therapist without sex therapy training is partially trained, as is a sex therapist without couples training.

As you will see in the following chapters, partners relentlessly vying for control can produce a wide variety of relationship-oriented symptoms. And while this may prove overwhelming to many clinicians, *Couples in Conflict* offers a broad approach to meet this challenge:

- Section I: Clinical Theory—In "Chapter 1. Introduction: Control and Conflict," control is defined as an internalized, paradoxical concept in which each partner in a relationship both needs and rejects control. Referred to as a control versus out-of-control master conflict, the dynamic produced by such a conflict can be responsible for control struggles in a couple and any associated symptoms. "Chapter 2. The Origin of Control Struggles" demonstrates how contradictory verbal and behavioral messages from the family of origin can lead to control conflicts in adult relationships. Significant life experiences, especially traumas are also considered factors. "Chapter 3. The Unconscious Process of Mate Selection" offers the uniquely deterministic perspective that long-term partners choose to mate with those who have the same internal conflict. This way the couple can preserve their conflict and establish a formidable resistance for the couple's therapist to contend with. And "Chapter 4. Controlling Styles" examines some of the techniques that partners use to exert control over one another such as verbal threatening, blaming, emotional manipulation, physical control including physical and sexual abuse, and financial abuse. Techniques used by partners to avoid being controlled are also examined such as avoidance or distancing, dismissiveness, passive-aggressive behavior, and procrastination. The point is made that an internal conflict about control often renders most of these techniques somewhat powerless in the long term.
- Section II: Clinical Assessment—In "Chapter 5. Assessing Couples with Control Struggles," the therapist is shown how to assess, with the use of the genogram, control struggles in couples who are exhibiting nonsexual symptoms such as disagreements about finances, as well as sexual symptoms such as delayed ejaculation and female orgasmic disorder. This chapter also serves to demonstrate how to understand a couple's collusion in the maintenance of a control struggle, and the art of working with process and content simultaneously. The therapist-couple fit is also addressed.

- Section III: Clinical Treatment—In "Chapter 6. Treatment Techniques for Couples with Control Struggles," the clinician is taught how to win the battle for therapeutic structure using a 5-step treatment process. This is especially difficult when couples are engaged in a battle for control. Also offered are practical, clinical techniques for breaking a couple's gridlock and alleviating nonsexual and sexual symptoms. A variety of diversified case examples are included along with one that demonstrates how sex therapy exercises are integrated into the model. "Chapter 7. How the Couples Therapist Can Avoid Being Caught in a Control Struggle" offers many creative tips on how the therapist can avoid being caught in a control struggle and rendered therapeutically impotent. And "Chapter 8. Termination and Relapse Prevention" helps the clinician to determine the appropriate time to terminate treatment and offers several practical techniques on how to make termination a smooth and ethical transition. The concept of premature termination is explored in detail, as well as its impact on the couple's therapist. And finally, the importance of relapse prevention in helping to maintain appropriate balance in a couple's control conflict is addressed.

Acknowledgements

My sincere appreciation to all the couples who have courageously allowed me to enter the inner sanctum of their relationships. It is hard to face the truth about oneself as an individual or as part of a couple, but it is the only reliable path to change.

Many thanks to my mentors and supervisors who have taught me the most challenging of all psychotherapies: couples therapy. They have instilled in me an unwavering confidence and passion.

—SJB

Section I

Clinical Theory

1 Introduction

Control and Conflict

One of the main objectives of this book is to demonstrate how two different, yet equally complex concepts—"control" and "conflict"—are inextricably linked in a way that can produce relationship gridlock and a host of associated symptoms, sexual and nonsexual. All partners struggle for control in their relationships at one time or another, but far too many couples are trapped in a vicious cycle competing for control. And while the struggle might sound straightforward enough, the concept is more complex.

Control Defined

Viorst (1998) defined control as: "The capacity to manage, dominate, exercise power over, influence, curb, suppress, or restrain" (p. 9). Here the concept of "control" is tailored specifically for relationships and defined as the ability to direct a partner's behavior. This may entail maneuvering them to behave in a particular way or to stop behaving in a way that is bothersome. While the concepts of power and control are related and often used interchangeably, I see the concept of power to be predominantly about dominance whereas control is more about a need-related, conflict driven anxiety. When two partners disagree with each other over an issue for an extended amount of time, and are unable to negotiate a compromise, they are in a control struggle. But there is much more to the concept of control as depicted by the following eight tenets:

1. **Chronic or fixed control struggles are problematic**: If control struggles are "fluid" or short-lived in a relationship, negotiation and compromise are more likely. Problems arise, however, when struggles for control become "fixed," or a couple is gridlocked over one or more significant issues. Here, the danger is that the battle for control may become the chief interactional process of the relationship with the couple stuck in an unproductive, often destructive cycle.
2. **Those who want control may also reject it**: Having control, a person feels safer and less anxious in part, because life is more predictable. To many, this form of equanimity is worth fighting for. But rarely is something that pure or simple, particularly when it comes to the complexity of interpersonal

DOI: 10.4324/9781003159100-2

relationships. If it were that easy, couples could routinely settle their differences and end their struggles. In my many years of exclusively treating couples with a wide variety of symptoms, I have found that those who strive for control are often simultaneously averse to it. This counterintuitive process suggests that each partner of a couple has an internal duality: control is both desired and paradoxically rejected.

3. **Striving for too much control may result in losing control:** A woman sought treatment because she could no longer tolerate her jealous, controlling husband's behavior: He would rarely let her out of the house. Despite pleas from his wife that she felt suffocated under his rule, he refused to relent. Then one day his greatest fear was realized: His wife confessed that she was engaged in an affair with a neighbor. Her defense was that because her husband refused to allow her more freedom, she had to take it for herself.

4. **Control exists on a continuum:** Like many concepts, control varies on a continuum with a strong need for control at one end and no pressing need for control on the other. Because partners will often assume control in specific areas, the more controlling a partner rates on the continuum, the more likely he/she is to bleed into the other's territory. Notice in Figure 1.1 that Jim is more controlling than Nancy, but less controlling than Tammy. Tammy is less controlling than Bill. Because Bill is clearly the closest to the extreme end of the continuum of control, he is most likely to try to take charge in all his relationships.

5. **People can, but typically do not exist at either extreme end of the control continuum:** In Figure 1.1 although Bill is more controlling than the others he is still not at the extreme end of the continuum. In fact, there is still room for someone else to be even more controlling. And while Nancy is the least controlling of all, she too is not at the extreme end, with room left for someone who is even less controlling. While one partner may be more controlling, the non-controller usually has "some" need for control and the controller has "some" need to be controlled or out-of-control. Rarely does a person completely reject any form or measure of control, especially in all contexts, and most controllers want a break from all their responsibilities.

Although one partner may have less of a need for control, what little this partner does take is usually expressed in a more passive or covert manner. So too, the controlling partner may give up control in the subtlest of ways. This paradox suggests an internal conflict that affords both partners—to varying degrees and intensity—a need for control and a need to be out-of-control (Betchen, 2010; Betchen & Davidson, 2018). This might also explain why some controlling

Noncontrolling_____Nancy_____Jim_____Tammy_____Bill_____Extremely Controlling

Figure 1.1   Control Continuum.

people appear to form relationships with those that are out-of-control and *vice versa*, thus creating the illusion of a unidimensional union.

Consider a woman with obsessive compulsive disorder (OCD) who marries an alcoholic. She may look as if she is the controlling partner. But can anyone really control an alcoholic? Or a rigid man who marries a woman with untreated attention-deficit/hyperactivity disorder (ADHD). This man may appear to be the organized, dominant force in the relationship, but is he really in control given the chaos his partner often brings to the union? While the Dominatrix works hard to maintain the "suspension of disbelief" in roleplaying the powerful figure in control of a BDSM process, most are quick to remind us that the client chooses, and pays for the fantasy (Betchen, 2014).

6. **The need for control transcends context:** Partners tend to assume control in specific areas. But some partners—those on the extreme end of the continuum of control—feel the need to control everyone and everything around them. These people are easier to recognize in treatment but less flexible and less likely to change.

7. **Control struggles can transcend age, gender, sexual orientation, culture, race, and socioeconomic status:** Any couple can engage in a battle for control and become gridlocked. These factors may be the cause of the struggle or may exacerbate it. This will be addressed throughout the remainder of the book.

8. **Control struggles are predominately born out of conflicts which emanate from each partner's family of origin:** As illustrated in Figure 1.2, these conflicts are then replicated in various ways and to varying degrees in adult relationships. Some children are raised in controlling households with rigid boundaries and strict limits. But I have found that these same households are permissive in counterintuitive ways. For example, Dana, from the time she was a child through her teen years, followed a rigid schedule of study, music lessons, and chores. She was forbidden to have playtime as a young girl, or to go to parties as a teen if it interfered with her responsibilities—no exceptions. But when Dana got her first boyfriend, her parents allowed him to sleep with Dana, in her bed. Even Dana was bewildered by her parents' permissiveness in this context.

As adults, individuals like Dana tend to replicate this conflict in their own families: modeling rigidity but with a component of permissiveness. Others with the same experience may choose the opposite environment in adulthood, erring towards permissiveness with a subtle hint of rigidity. The replication process depends largely on the child's nature and perspective. For example, if a young boy saw his beloved father constantly persecuted by the boy's mother, as an adult he might decide to role model his father's responses, but simultaneously retain his mother's need to persecute. Alternately, he may try to make sure this never happens to him by identifying with his mother's power while in less obvious ways, absorbing his father's need for persecution.

Treatment

(Master Conflict Therapy)

Nonsexual---Symptoms---Sexual

Control Struggles

(Master Conflict: Control vs. Out-of-Control)

Internal Conflict ----------------- Internal Conflict

Family of Origin -----------------Family of Origin

Partner #1 ----------------------- Partner #2

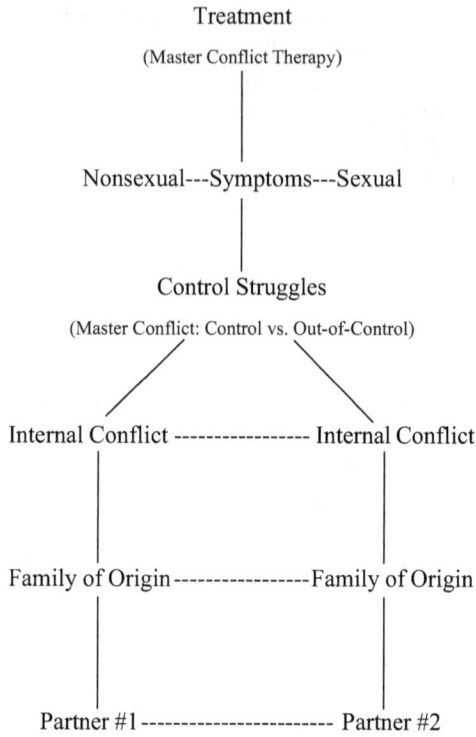

Figure 1.2   The Origin of Control.

In my clinical experience, I have found that if one grows up in a family of origin that struggles with control, it will be hard to avoid replicating control struggles in adult relationships. Remarkably, these individuals also may choose a life partner who also has a conflict around control, supporting Bowen's (1978) *multigenerational transmission process*. This will be discussed in greater detail in "Chapter 2. The Origin of Control Struggles."

Internal Conflict

When couples therapists use the word conflict, they are generally referring to a disagreement or fight "between" two partners. This *external conflict* is reflected in the couple's overt symptoms and is therefore easy for the couple's therapist to recognize. Because of its visibility, it may even be relatively easy to determine what the couple are fighting about; or at least what they think they are fighting about.

Most couples who seek treatment present in turmoil, or conflict in the traditional sense of the word, and sometimes they can be quite volatile. They can also prove chaotic and dominate the therapeutic process. But no matter how challenging, the couple is exposing their dynamic in real time giving the therapist a picture of what life outside the session is like. Rarely can a couple compartmentalize well enough to appear completely different in a different context.

An *internal conflict*, however, is often much more difficult to comprehend. It is as if two opposing parts of the self are having an ongoing argument with no acceptable solution. Even more confusing, because an internal conflict is wholly beyond our awareness, it is difficult to directly correlate it to any symptoms. For example, Tom's mother constantly chided him to do his chores and punished him severely for disobeying. Because of this, he internalized a conflict about pleasing her: part of him wanted to meet with her approval and stop her from berating him; the other part of him wanted to rebel and frustrate her—to show her he cannot be pushed around. Tom's wife Deborah unknowingly triggered her husband's conflicted feelings towards his mother and he in turn transferred these feelings onto his wife. This baffled Deborah because she thought their argument was literally about something as simple as taking out the trash. She had no idea that in Tom's mind, she has taken on the role of her husband's demanding mother figure.

People may be aware of one part of their internal conflict but not both parts. For example, Tom might be conscious of his desire to make Deborah happy and to stop her attacks, but unaware of his need to anger and frustrate her—to do battle with her; or his need to pick chronically dissatisfied women. He keeps the latter part of the conflict hidden from himself because the complete truth reveals the unpleasant and unadmirable part of the self. And while he may put an end to the madness in his relationship, he will most likely pay a price: He may have to give up battling his mother and emotionally accept her as she is. Quite a price to pay.

Deborah is aware that her husband is letting her down by not doing his share of the chores—this is her main complaint. But she may not be conscious of her desire to render Tom impotent, or her tendency to choose men who fail to meet her needs. To face this side of herself, she may need to confront a fear she has of becoming like her weak father. The following exchange illustrates this dynamic:

Deborah: I can't ask you to do anything for me. If it's important to me, you never seem to care enough.

Tom: That's not true. I always want to please you. I just think you're never satisfied.

Deborah: Name a time you did what I've asked you to do. If you want to please me so bad there must be plenty of them.

Tom: I can't think of anything right now. But I know that I've done a lot of things for you, and I do want to make you happy. Do you really think I enjoy being yelled at all the time?

Deborah: But you can't even come up with one example.

Tom: Okay, two weeks ago, you asked me to take off from work to help you fix the garage door and I did it even though I was under stress at work.

Deborah: Well, it's your garage door too.

Tom: That's what I am talking about.

Deborah: And what about the times I've asked you to help put the kids to bed, or go grocery shopping, or help me with the bills? Where were you then? Sometimes I do not even know why I got married.

Tom: Whatever I do doesn't matter because you'll never be satisfied with me.

Both partners were right about each other: Tom did little for Deborah, and his primary excuse was that she was impossible to please. Deborah proved Tom correct by responding negatively to the one thing he did do for her: fix the garage door. But neither partner saw their complete selves—an unfortunate circumstance because without personal insight, neither could see both sides of their respective conflict and take personal responsibility for the continuing demise of their relationship.

Because of its amorphous nature, it is much more difficult to convince individuals that they might have an internal conflict. And because it is also counterintuitive, most people have a difficult time accepting that they may be doing something to prevent the stated achievement of their goals. It also suggests a lack of free will, or that something inside is determining their behavior.

I am not the first to consider internal conflict as the source of external symptoms. Freud (1910/1957) saw conflict as a battle between instinctual drives and opposing forces. He proposed two potential solutions to this struggle: to negotiate a compromise between the two or to sublimate the drive. Freud warned that the solution requires the frustration of one of these forces at the expense of the other.

Fairbairn (1952/1986), developer of the *Object Relations* model, contended that the origin of conflict began with a child's conflict between the good versus bad parts of their idealized primary caregiver—usually the mother. To defend against accepting the bad parts of the mother, the child internalizes and loses these parts in the self. Dicks (1967) and Scharff and Scharff (1994) have applied this approach to working with couples.

In the *Theory of Neurotic Needs*, Horney (1945/1966) wrote that the seat of neurosis ultimately was in a child's ability to cope with the conflicts that arise among three tendencies: moving towards (compliance), moving against (aggression), and moving away from people (withdrawal). Healthy people can move in any one of these directions at any time, but conflicted people have difficulty.

More recently, some systems therapists have contended that internal conflict is responsible for various psychological symptoms. For example, in the *Internal Family Systems (IFS)* approach developed by Schwartz (1997), the author contends that people have sub-personalities or parts of self, and that these parts interact the way people do, except they do so internally, not externally. The sub-personalities are often in conflict with one another and with one's core self, a concept that describes the confident, compassionate, whole person, which is at the core of every person. The objective of IFS is to heal the wounded parts and restore mental balance by changing the dynamics that create discord among the sub-personalities and the self (Schwartz & Sweezy, 2020).

The Master Conflict

The model used in this book to treat internal conflict is referred to as Master Conflict Therapy (MCT). MCT is an integrative, psychodynamic, systems model developed (Betchen, 2010) and refined (Betchen & Davidson, 2018; Betchen & Gambescia, 2020) specifically to treat diverse couples who suffer from a variety of relationship problems, including sexual disorders. The basic premise of MCT is that each partner shares one conflict that is primarily responsible for most of the couple's significant relationship symptoms, hence the term "master conflict." While they may have many smaller conflicts, the couple's master conflict is the deepest, most powerful, and most pervasive conflict; and yet, it is partly hidden from them. That is, they may be aware of one side of the conflict but not the other.

A master conflict is an internal duality: two opposing parts of the self that compete against one another to direct our emotions and behaviors from within. One example might be that a part of you has a need to be financially successful, but the other part fails to see the value in this endeavor. From an operational perspective, one part insists on pushing you to take on new and promising projects and to increase your stature, but the other part takes a more relaxed approach and may in fact sabotage your efforts or any success you have achieved.

Throughout a relationship, the two internalized sides may vacillate with little problem. But when one side attempts to dominate the other, the master conflict is said to be unbalanced and relationship symptoms usually appear. For example, if one side pursues a certain modicum of success but makes some room for moderation and *vice versa*, the conflict is said to be balanced. But if one side attempts to dominate the other, it is imbalanced.

One or both partners can unbalance a master conflict at any time if either of them try to change the set dynamics of their master conflict. For example, if one decides to be more, or less successful than agreed upon. For the most part, however because partners choose each other based on having the same master conflict (see "Chapter 3. The Unconscious Process of Mate Selection"), they generally reinforce their shared conflict.

You would think it might be less complicated if partners could simply choose one part of the conflict over the other, but both sides have enough merit, making it too close of a call. For example, driving yourself to succeed is a worthy cause, but you may have to give up certain freedoms or even suffer losses, such as a neglected spouse, to reach your objective. On the other hand, if you work less, you might be less stressed, but you will accumulate less material goods, and have less stature in your community. Simply put, you will have to give up something to get something no matter which side you take, and this is not what most of us want to hear. No one wants to suffer loss of any kind, and for this reason alone people will choose the paralysis of the conflict over risking the anxiety that comes from whatever lies ahead or the depression that often accompanies whatever is left behind.

Choosing a side may also prove futile because the rejected side will always exist within you anyway; it will always have to be reckoned with in varying degrees. This is not to say that master conflicts are naturally bad or pathological because they do exist in even the healthiest of couples. But they can be devastatingly problematic when unbalanced. The key then is not to side with one part of the master conflict over the other, but to balance the conflict by integrating the two parts in a way that is most comfortable to each partner and the couple. This will be addressed in detail in "Chapter 6. Treatment and Techniques for Couples with Control Struggles."

To illustrate this dynamic, I often use the metaphor of an internal seesaw with two politicians—one on each side—arguing a point deftly enough so that we cannot seem to choose who to believe (Betchen, 2010; Betchen & Davidson, 2018). If a master conflict is balanced enough, neither side of the seesaw will be up too high or too low for an extended period—the couple will usually be symptom free. Only when one side of the conflict dominates for too long a period (one side of the seesaw is either too far up or down), are they are said to be unbalanced. If a couple agree not to have sex, for example, and have not had any for years, their shared master conflict, whichever one it is, is said to be balanced. This happens when each partner's master conflict is in sync. But if one becomes set on having sex, the relational equilibrium in this context is unbalanced and may cause a problem, especially if the other partner refuses.

Notice in Figure 1.3, the master conflict depicted by a seesaw is balanced because both partners agree not to buy a new house. In Figure 1.4, the seesaw is quite off balance because only one partner wants a new house. Again, if this imbalance lasts at this level and with this intensity, the couple will have serious problems. If the seesaw soon swings back in balance or stabilizes, the couple can recover and live harmoniously with their conflict. In Figure 1.5 the couple reach a reasonably comfortable compromise on when to buy a new house.

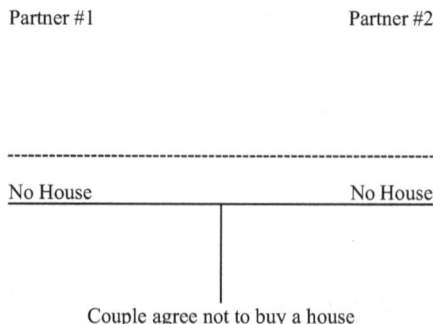

Partner #1   Partner #2

No House   No House

Couple agree not to buy a house

Figure 1.3   Balanced Master Conflict.

Partner #1   Partner #2

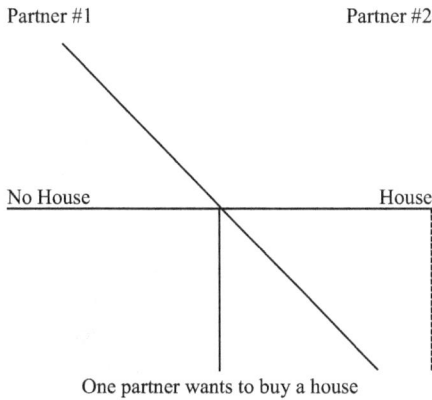

No House   House

One partner wants to buy a house

Figure 1.4   Unbalanced Master Conflict.

Partner #1   Partner #2

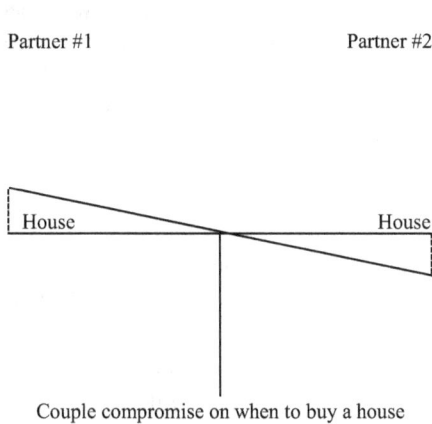

House   House

Couple compromise on when to buy a house

Figure 1.5   Comfortable Balance of Master Conflict.

The Control Versus Out-of-Control Master Conflict

In previous work I have identified 19 different master conflicts that if unbalanced may plague couples. I have pointed out that while each couple has their "one and only" specific master conflict, other couples may have the same one or any one of the other 19 conflicts. Here I focus on the master conflict that I have determined to be the most pervasive and potentially damaging to a couple—the one that presents a formidable challenge to most couples therapists: *control versus out-of-control* (Betchen, 2010; Betchen & Davidson, 2018). In this conflict, one part of each partner feels a strong need to be in control; the other part experiences an equally strong need to be out-of-control or controlled by the behavior of others. A common example of this is the enabler and a sexually addicted or sexual compulsive partner. The enabler works hard to curb or control his/her partner's behavior, while the addict continues to create chaos. Why would a controlling person partner up with someone so out-of-control?

Why would someone who craves chaos partner with a controlling person? While each partner claims to detest one side of their respective counterpart, they crave the other. The enabler needs something to try and control, and the addict desperately needs the enabler's structure. While the matchup often fails, these partners are drawn to each other and the process itself proves to be magnetic. Many women formerly married to addicts have an admittedly hard time adjusting to a life without battle—perhaps the battle to rehabilitate someone. Once they begin to date nonaddicts they often claim to be bored; many even lose their sex drive. What they are suggesting is that a life free of battle is uncomfortable to them.

I have found—in my many years of studying couples in conflict—that battles for control are responsible for myriad relational symptoms, as well as numerous breakups. There is a reason why when most couples divorce, they cite: "irreconcilable differences." And the reason is not always because partners wish to avoid laying blame and inflaming the process. The term is often used as a vague, mutual accusation that is euphemistic for implacable control struggles. In her book *Imperfect Control*, Viorst (1998) wrote: "Weak or strong, man or woman, we can't be in a close relationship without attempting to exercise control" (p. 130). The following example depicts a control struggle with the context being their children's education:

Nicole: I think it's ridiculous to send our kids to expensive colleges. They will do just as well to attend state colleges, which are less than half the price of fancy Ivy League schools.

Kurt: We've been arguing about this since the kids were in the 7th grade. I agree that it will stretch us financially. But I want the best for our kids and going to better colleges will give them an advantage. Besides, if they do well enough to get into great schools how can we limit their choices?

Nicole: You better learn how to limit them or that ulcer you once had will come back. Personally, I don't want the stress.

Kurt: (Raising his voice) I think arguing with you was the cause of my ulcer.

Nicole: Can we just agree to disagree?

Kurt: We can't do that. We need a plan. If we stay away from the Ivies, can we at least agree to some schools just beneath them?

Nicole: No, state colleges it is. If they want to take out enormous loans for graduate or professional school that's on them. I want to be able to sleep at night. And besides, we both went to state schools and did fine.

Kurt: I want my kids to do better than us. It's why I work so hard.

As is so often the case with control struggles, notice that neither Kurt nor Nicole is necessarily wrong when it comes to the future of their children's education. Both partners make convincing arguments to support their positions. And if you polled ten couples they might split evenly on this subject. But because the partners were not on the same page—and have never been so—they experience marital difficulty. In this case, there was a growing tension which eventually infiltrated their sex lives, and the couple eventually divorced citing a difference in values. If they were more fluid in their approach to the problem, they might have been able to stay married. To revisit my old metaphor, the couple's seesaw was completely unbalanced.

The remainder of this book endeavors to help professional couples therapists—who work with couples of all races, ethnicities, and sexual orientation—recognize the complexity and contradictions of control struggles, determine their origins, understand how these struggles may be responsible for their symptoms, and to break these destructive patterns to alleviate their associated symptoms.

Sociocultural Context

A discussion about the general concept of control would not be complete without considering it in the context of sociocultural factors. Historically, male-dominated rules have controlled women's behavior. In early America, for example, the legal document of marital unity was referred to as a *coverture* and the wife, a *feme covert*. "Coverture in its strictest sense of the word meant that a wife could not use legal avenues such as suits or contracts, own assets, or execute legal documents without her husband's collaboration" (Cott, 2000, p. 11). Women were not even allowed to keep property they owned prior to marriage (Salmon, 1986). Cott (2000) claimed that the husband was the "one *full* citizen in the household, his authority over and responsibility for his dependents contributing to his citizen capacity" (p. 12). According to Hartog (2000), "the law made a wife into a 'thing,' a 'nonentity,' a 'slave'" (p. 122).

While men were in control of the family finances and made major decisions for all family members, women did have their roles: Women took care of household and family duties such as cooking and cleaning. They also served as nurturers and caregivers, and the primary parent of the children. Unmarried women often carried similar obligations in someone else's household (Lewis, 2019). There was little overlap in these roles and each partner was to do his/her job to maintain the functional flow of the family system. And while couples still experienced control struggles, each partner was somewhat limited by context in his/her ability to exert control. For example, if a woman became angry with her husband her primary means of expressing it might have been withholding affection or falling short on family duties. A man might have restricted his wife's finances.

The prospects for women began to see some improvement courtesy of the Women's Rights Movement of the mid-1800s and the Civil Rights Movement of the 1960s. Subsequently, the jostle for gender equality has continued to incrementally improve, and with it, those once rigid traditional roles have become somewhat blurred. It is no longer a guarantee that a man alone will even be able to support a family. And a narrowing of the gender gap in education, employment, and pay has led, in some couples, to a role reversal—unthinkable in early America.

We are now witness to many female breadwinners coupled with men who assume a significant amount of responsibility for domestic affairs. Although women still average an hour more of housework per day, men have doubled their time spent on housework since 1965 (Donner, 2020). Approximately 85% of women and 71% percent of men spend some time each day doing housework, cooking, lawn care, or household management (U.S. Bureau of Labor Statistics, 2020).

The Pew Research Center reports that females now make up 47% of the workforce in the United States, up from 30% in 1950. Women in heterosexual relationships now comprise approximately 31% of the breadwinner roles in their families (Geiger & Parker, 2018) and women's earnings have risen at a greater rate than men's earnings, by 45%, from $15 in 1980 to $22 in 2018 (Kochhar, 2020). A gender pay gap still does exist, however: The US Bureau of Labor Statistics (2020) reported that the median weekly salary for full-time female workers is $902 or 81.7% of the $1,104 for men. White females had a median weekly income of $910 while Black and Hispanic females averaged $768 and $722, respectively.

Couples therapists—most of whom are women—support gender equality but are objective enough to admit there is a price. They acknowledge that because white, heterosexual men have long been in control, learning to share it has not been easy. Gander (2018) found that loss of control has even led to an increase in male aggression towards women. The #MeToo movement has been an effort to call attention to the sexual abuse and other forms of discrimination many women face at the hands of powerful men, especially as these women compete for equality in the workplace. The movement advances the notion that sexual harassment should be considered by the public community as a health issue with implications for disease prevention and health promotion (O'Neil et al., 2018).

Studies, however, show that women are not exactly acclimated to being in control in nontraditional areas nor do many want to be. Anti-feminists notwithstanding, according to Tinsely (2015), Americans across gender and race still favor male breadwinners. Ford (2017) reported that even millennial women are in conflict when they out earn their male partners. Such change and confusion may be responsible for the increased number of couples in control struggles entering my clinical practice. And because this dynamic is a potentially destructive process, a couple can exhibit a variety of symptoms, sexual and nonsexual.

Same-sex couples are said to have more egalitarian relationships (Green, 2014; Perales & Baxter, 2017) and yet they too, battle for control at times. Howard (2016) found that gay men are subjected to the "masculine ideal" which may breed intense competition for breadwinner status. And with a rise in the number of intermarriages between people of different races and ethnicities (Geiger & Livingston, 2019), sociocultural differences will no doubt lend themselves to new sets of control struggles.

Our country is divided as sections of it battle along partisan lines. Current events have fueled the fire and political controversy has reached a high pitch.

Disagreements over these macro issues have infiltrated the family home, creating a wider context for couples to engage in control struggles (Betchen, 2020a). One client reported that she was leaving her husband because she "can't stand his politics."

We also have a virus (Covid-19) that is highly contagious, causing couples to spend exponentially more time together. Sheltering in place for months together has shined a light on pre-existing tensions that might have ordinarily been avoided or repressed (Betchen, 2020b). One man, who for years traveled internationally for business, said that he knew that his wife was controlling, but never realized just how much. This led him to ask her, tongue in cheek: "Gee, how did I ever survive before I met you."

References

Betchen, S. (2010). *Magnetic partners: Discover how the hidden conflict that once attracted you to each other is now driving you apart*. Free Press.

Betchen, S. (2014, December 25). Sexually dominant women and the men who desire them: Part III. *Psychology Today*. www.psychologytoday.com/us/blog/magnetic-partners/201412/sexually-dominant-women-and-the-men-who-desire-them-part-iii

Betchen, S. (2020a, June 27). When couples fight about politics. *Psychology Today*. www.psychologytoday.com/us/blog/magnetic-partners/202006/when-couples-fight-about-politics

Betchen, S. (2020b, April 8). Love in the time of coronavirus. *Psychology Today*. www.psychologytoday.com/us/blog/magnetic-partners/202004/love-in-the-time-coronavirus

Betchen, S., & Davidson, H. (2018). *Master conflict therapy: A new model for practicing couples and sex therapy*. Routledge.

Betchen, S., & Gambescia, N. (2020). A new systemic treatment model for couples with premature ejaculation: Master conflict theory. In K. Hertlein, N. Gambescia, & G. Weeks (Eds.), *Systemic sex therapy* (3rd ed., pp. 77–91). Routledge.

Bowen, M. (1978). *Family therapy in clinical practice*. Aronson.

Cott, N. (2000). *Public vows: A history of marriage and the nation*. Harvard University Press.

Dicks, H.V. (1967). *Marital tensions: Clinical studies towards a psychological theory of interaction*. Karnac Books.

Donner, F. (2020, February 12). The household work men and women do, and why. *NYTimes*. www.nytimes.com/2020/02/12/us/the-household-work-men-women-do-and-why.html

Fairbairn, W.R.D. (1952/1986). *Psychoanalytic studies of the personality*. Routledge.

Ford, A. (2017, May 1). *Millennial women are conflicted about being breadwinners*. Refinery29. www.refinery29.com/en-us/2017/04/148488/millennial-women-are-conflicted-about-being-breadwinners

Freud, S. (1910/1957). Five lectures on psycho-analysis, Leonardo da Vinci and other works. In J. Strachey (Ed. and Trans.), *The standard edition of the complete psychological works of Sigmund Freud* (Vol. 11., pp. 9–238). Hogarth Press and the Institute for Psycho-analysis.

Gander, K. (2018, November 26). Sexist men get aggressive when they think women want to control them: Study. *Newsweek: Tech & Science*. www.newsweek.com/sexist-men-get-aggressive-when-they-think-women-want-control-them-study-1230657

Geiger, A.W., & Livingston, G. (2019, February 13). *8 facts about love and marriage in America*. Pew Research Center. www.pewresearch.org/fact-tank/2019/02/13/8-facts-about-love-and-marriage/

Geiger, A.W., & Parker, K. (2018, March 15). *For women's history month, a look at gender gains- and gaps-in the U.S.* Pew Research Center. www.pewresearch.org/facttank/2018/03/15/ for-women's-history-month-a-look-at-gender-gains-and-gaps-in-the-u-s/

Green, R.-J. (2014, December 29). *Same-sex couples may have more egalitarian relationships* [Interview]. National Public Radio; Alliant International University. www.alliant.edu/blog/ professor-emeritus-dr-robert-jay-green-same-sex-couples-may-have-more-egalitarian

Hartog, H. (2000). *Man & wife in America: A history*. Harvard University Press.

Horney, K. (1945/1966). *Our inner conflicts*. Norton.

Howard, K. (2016, July 24). Gay men's relationships: 10 ways they differ from straight relationships. *HuffPost*. www.huffpost.com/entry/gay-mens-relationships-ten-ways-they-differ-from_b_57950dd0e4b0b3e2427c9022

Kochhar, R. (2020, January 30). *Women's lead in skills and education is helping narrow the gender wage*. Pew Research Center. www.pewsocialtrends.org/2020/01//30/ womens-lead-in-skills-and-education-is-hewlping-narrow-the-gender-gap/

Lewis, J.J. (2019, September 11). *Women and work in early America*. ThoughtCo. www. thoughtco.com/women-at-work-early-america-3530833

O'Neil, A., Sojo, V., Fileborn, B., Scovelle, A., & Milner, A. (2018). The #MeToo movement: An opportunity in public health. *Lancet, 391*, 2587–2589. https://doi.org/10.1016/ S0140-6736(18)30991-7

Perales, F., & Baxter, J. (2017). Sexual identity and relationship quality in Australia and the United Kingdom. *Family Relations, 67*, 55–69. https://doi.org/10.11/fare.12293

Salmon, M. (1986). *Women and the law of property in early America*. University of North Carolina Press.

Scharff, D., & Scharff, J. (1994). *Object relations couple therapy*. Aronson.

Schwartz, R. (1997). *Internal family systems therapy*. Guilford.

Schwartz, R., & Sweezy, M. (2020). *Internal family systems therapy* (2nd ed.). Guilford.

Tinsely, C. (2015, March 23). *Primary breadwinners should be men, majority of Americans say*. Georgetown University. www.georgetown.edu/news/primary-breadwinners-should-be-men-majority-of-americans-say/

U.S. Bureau of Labor Statistics (2020). *American time use survey summary*. U.S. Department of Labor. Retrieved July 22, 2021, from www.bls.gov/tus/

Viorst, J. (1998). *Imperfect control*. Free Press.

2   The Origin of Control Struggles

Conflicts about control usually emanate from two major sources: (1) the family of origin; and (2) certain intense life experiences, specifically trauma. According to Bowen (1978), our families leave an indelible mark on us that can be managed, but never completely erased. Toman (1976) wrote: "A person's family represents the most influential context of his life, and it exerts its influence more regularly, more exclusively, and earlier in a person's life than do any other life contexts" (p, 5). Seemingly harmless messages from the family of origin, if conveyed consistently, can serve to steer our lives in directions we might not have otherwise chosen.

"Psychological trauma has developed into a very common concept in the scientific community, in mental healthcare, as well as in popular language and mass media" (Kleber, 2019, p. 1). Trauma has been found to be responsible for a host of psychological symptoms such as anxiety and depression, and physical symptoms like chronic fatigue, autoimmune diseases, and substance abuse (van der Kolk, 2014). You do not have to have fought in a war to experience trauma; other events can have a similar impact on our lives such as natural disasters, the death of a loved one, or experiencing family violence, to name a few.

The Family of Origin

As children we are subjected to verbal (e.g., words), and nonverbal (e.g., body language) messages in our families of origin. While some of these messages convey a singular meaning, a second, contradictory message also may be conveyed, creating confusion. This second message may be delivered either simultaneously or soon after the original message. A contradictory message may be verbal, nonverbal, or a combination of both. This is what communication experts refer to as a "metamessage." Tannen (2011) wrote: "Information conveyed by the meanings of words is the message. What is communicated about relationships—attitude towards each other, the occasion, and what we are saying—is the metamessage" (p. 29). As will be demonstrated in "Section II. Clinical Assessment," a pattern of specific metamessages can lead the clinician to the source of a couple's internal conflict.

DOI: 10.4324/9781003159100-3

A child may begin to develop an internal conflict around control if one or both parents habitually conveyed mixed messages about control. The more direct and frequently communicated, and the more significant the context, the greater the chance for internalization. In my many years of clinical practice I have noticed three predominant ways that these messages are delivered: (1) contradictory messages from one parent—one parent is responsible for conveying mixed messages while the other parent takes a neutral or passive stance; (2) contradictory messages from both parents—each parent delivers the same message and in doing so they form a dysfunctional, united front; and (3) parents with opposing messages—each parent communicates a different or opposing message. The danger here is that it often forces the child to choose sides.

Contradictory Messages From One Parent

Tom and Sara were a couple in their early 30s who presented for treatment because they were fighting over Tom's career path. Tom wanted to work for the family contracting business, but Sara was not fond of the owner: her father-in-law, Jim. Jim founded the business and built it into the success it eventually became. Ever since he was a small boy, Tom remembered that Jim talked about turning over the business to him when he retired. According to Tom, Jim had routinely bragged about how smart and capable Tom was.

True to his word, approximately five years before he was to retire, Jim brought Tom into the business to teach him what he would need to make the transition smooth. But once there, Jim gave Tom little responsibility. Tom claimed that he had nothing to do, and whenever he came up with a business-related idea his father would ignore it; sometimes he would roll his eyes and dismiss Tom with a wave of his hand. On other occasions, Jim would simply tell Tom that his idea was silly.

Tom did not know what to do, but his wife Sara did. She put enormous pressure on Tom to leave the family business and build his career elsewhere. Sara said that she did not think Jim would ever turn over control to anyone. But Tom was reluctant to sever ties with the family business; it was a lucrative enterprise that promised security for he and his family. The couple were gridlocked in a control struggle about whether to stay or leave the family business.

I got a bird's eye view of Tom's dilemma when, with Tom and Sara's permission, I honored Jim's request for a session with he and his wife, Carol. Apparently, Tom let his father know that he was not happy with their current business arrangement and his father was confused. Consider the following exchange:

Jim: We hear you're the best around.

Therapist: Psychotherapy is a subjective experience.

Jim: Did you read all those books on your shelves?

Therapist: With the help of cliff notes.

Jim: (Chuckles) Listen before you say anything, I have a couple of questions to ask you.

Therapist: Okay.

Jim: How long is this going to take? Some of you guys keep people in here forever.

Therapist: You asked for the session.

Jim: I know. But I just hope you are not thinking of blaming my wife and I for Tom's problems.

Therapist: I wouldn't dream of it.

Jim: What is my son's problem? He doesn't seem to be getting any better.

Therapist: I appreciate your concerns. But I think I can better help your family if I can find out a little more about you and your wife.

Carol: Dear, let him ask us some questions. Doctor, Jim is used to being the boss.

It is not hard to see why Tom is having trouble working for his father. Jim was clearly trying to control the treatment. He told me that I was the best, but he blocked me from doing my work. Like he did with his son, he tried not to allow me to have any control. He did most of the talking, rarely leaving any space for Carol or me to get a word in. He also peppered me with questions and in this way tried to keep me on the defensive.

Carol intervened only after several minutes and was careful in doing so. She even offered an excuse for her husband's behavior. I determined from her relative passivity that she was no help to Tom. With such a controlling father and weak mother, Tom had little chance to feel confident on a personal level and to gain any control in the family business. Jim gave Tom mixed messages most of Tom's life: he was both competent and incompetent. Once revealed, Tom began to remember several examples in which his father failed to promote his competence.

Tom was in a control struggle with Sara over his career choice, but they also fought about sex—arguing about frequency and quality. It could be said with confidence that Tom has spent most of his life engaged in one or more control struggles. As mentioned, partners share the same internal master conflict. It would then follow that Sara would have a conflict about control as well. Even though she was probably right about Tom's father, she presented as rigid and controlling. She expressed her point of view but rarely left any space for Tom. In her single-parent family of origin, Sara was parentified (Boszormenyi-Nagy & Spark, 1973). She not only held down two jobs—one in a supermarket and another as a receptionist—but was also charged with taking care of her two younger siblings. It was she, not her mother, who raised her siblings, and it was she who was called upon to help her mother make major-life decisions. Sara was trained from a young age to take control and she did so dutifully.

Contradictory Messages From Unified Parents

Craig and Jenna were a couple in their late 30s. The couple reported for treatment because Jenna felt Craig used her as a "sexual object." She said Craig insisted that she have sex with him whenever he wanted, but he showed little affection or tenderness towards her. When Craig demanded that Jenna perform certain sexual acts, she drew the line and threatened to stop having sex altogether unless Craig agreed to go for couples therapy. Craig held out for several months, but he gave in and accompanied Jenna to treatment. Craig and Jenna had other control struggles as well: They disagreed over finances and the disciplining of the children. Apparently, Craig had a heavy hand while Jenna was too permissive. And while they differed on many things, they each shared a background of control struggles. The following example depicts their immediate struggle:

Craig: Jenna doesn't like sex. She doesn't even fantasize.

Jenna: I like it. But I won't do some of the kinky things you want me to do.

Craig: Lots of people do these things. I'm not weird. You're just uptight.

Jenna: No, I'm not. I just find some of those things disgusting. You get plenty of sex. You don't need more.

Craig: Let's ask the doctor. Do you think I'm being unreasonable?

Therapist: What I think doesn't matter. You two are not on the same page, and you've been stuck on this issue for so long it is spilling over into other areas of your life together.

It is obvious that Craig and Jenna are locked into a control struggle with sex as the chief complaint. Jenna refuses to give in to Craig's desires, and Craig cannot give up on the possibility that she will one day give in. He has been pestering Jenna for some time and she is getting fed up. Craig has used several tactics to weaken Jenna's stance on the matter—he even resorted to diagnosing her as "uptight." But he did not try to negotiate with her. While she may not have compromised, Craig did not give her the opportunity. Consider each partner's family of origin to find out where their controlling tendencies come from.

Craig was one of three brothers raised in a large family furniture business run by his father and mother. This business was successful enough to support Craig and many of his siblings and their families. Craig, like Tom from the previous case, was told he would one day soon have an executive role in the business. But unlike Tom, he was promised this by "both" parents. He was also encouraged to pursue, and to take what he wanted in life—a message that inspired a lot of brutal competition between he and his siblings. However, after Craig's father passed unexpectedly, his mother took complete control over the business, citing her many control struggles with her husband. She was now in charge and had no plans to elevate Craig.

Craig stayed with the company for a few more years battling his mother, but his efforts proved fruitless. He finally saw no other option but to give up and leave the company. Craig had to face reality after his father passed: His parents were always a united front, ruling their company with an iron fist. Nobody came between the two and Craig's mother was slated to take the company over all along.

Jenna's mother was sickly most of her life from various forms of cancer and Jenna was her caretaker. Like Sara, she was parentified (Boszormenyi-Nagy & Spark, 1973) but more severely. Her father was very passive and heavily relied on Jenna to help with her mother, take care of her younger siblings, and to give him emotional support. While both Jenna's parents made it clear to Jenna that she was to run the family, they were rarely satisfied with her efforts; they in fact often rebelled against her decisions and methods.

Both Jenna's parents demanded that Jenna work harder to please her mother, and yet they fought Jenna on everything related to her mother's healthcare even though Jenna was acting on doctor's orders. When Jenna appealed to her father to intervene, he would refuse. He told Jenna to simply try even harder to make his sickly wife happy—an impossible task. He said that he did not want her to upset his wife at all costs. Jenna was confused. Her parents claimed to give her control of the family but undermined her every move. She was both in control and not in control. Jenna soon rebelled and began to find reasons to stay out of the house.

In response to Jenna's distance, both parents increased their demands on Jenna. She in turn became more passive aggressive. Jenna would: forget to buy certain food requested by her mother; neglect to regiment her mother's medication; fail to run errands; burn meals; and let dirty dishes pile up. In this sense, she allowed her parents less and less control over her life.

Craig was physically attracted to Jenna from the start, but it was the couple's mutual conflict about control that truly bonded them. If you recall, Craig was raised by aggressive parents who taught him to take what he wanted, and he wanted Jenna; so, he aggressively pursued her. Jenna, always the reluctant pleaser, gave in to his whims until she got fed up and rebelled. For example, Craig tried to take what he wanted sexually. He relentlessly pursued Jenna for sex but the harder he pushed the more resistance he encountered.

While Craig tried to be in control, his efforts led to less control. Jenna gave into her husband for a time but found him impossible to satisfy, just as she did her parents. And just as she did as a young parentified child, she eventually stopped trying to please. The couple stayed locked into a control struggle for years until Jenna finally put up a roadblock that Craig could not blast through. The couple were in gridlock.

Parents Who Contradict Each Other

Gary and Rita were a married couple in their 50s who historically disagreed about many things such as how many children to have and where to live. But their primary problem was a control struggle over money. Gary was a spender and Rita was a saver. For many years, these struggles were limited to minor skirmishes but as both aged and the stakes grew higher, the couple became less amenable to negotiating. Finally, Rita was threatening to leave Gary. She claimed that without him she could have complete control over her finances. Gary did not want a divorce, but he was getting progressively tired of Rita's financial restrictions, which he saw as neurotic. Consider the following exchange:

Rita: I can't take it anymore. Every time we get ahead financially Gary comes up with a reason to spend what we have. I'm tired of stressing about money. I don't want to sit around waiting for his next big idea.

Gary: Rita thinks we are always on the verge of going broke. She'd prefer to stick every penny away and die with a boat load of money in the bank. What good is having money if we can't enjoy it? Besides, I'm not the spendthrift she makes me out to be. She's the cheapest person I know.

Therapist: Rita, it seems that Gary's style makes you anxious.

Rita: Yes, there are times that I can't even sleep at night. Maybe if "he" paid the bills he would see my point.

Gary: There's no need for that. I know how much we make because I make most of it. If we had $10,000,000 in the bank you'd still worry. You're just like your crazy parents when it comes to money; they still think another big depression is around the corner.

This is a good segue into each partner's family of origin. Rita was the oldest of three sisters. Her family was middle-class, but her parents grew up in the Great Depression. As a result, they instilled in their children that money and food were vital for survival. They had a distrust of banks and the stock market, and they stored away enough can goods to feed an army; they also kept several large freezers filled with food in their basement.

Rita was conscious of her parent's issues with money and how they impacted her childhood, but she considered their financial methods as somewhat sound. But while Rita's parents presented a unified front when it came to spending money in general, there was one major point of contention: Rita's father wanted to send Rita to college and graduate school and was willing to sacrifice to do so. Her mother, however, was adamantly against this; she saw it as an exorbitant waste of money. When Rita got into an Ivy League University, it created a huge rift between the parents with the mother eventually winning out.

Gary was the oldest of two siblings. His parents were hard-working people who agreed that it was important to enjoy life. But Gary's father spent more money than his wife would have liked. He also was not a saver. Gary's father lived for today and often said "you can't take it with you." Gary's mother was frugal and savvy with money. She often fought with her husband about many of his spending habits and financial decision-making, to no avail. Gary would chuckle and say that his parents had more fun in their lives than he and Rita would ever experience. But it did bother him that he would have to pay for his own college tuition as well as subsidize his parents in their old age; something Rita resented.

Rita's internalized conflict with control was evident in the context of money. She was terrified of being poor but would use her money for what she deemed practical—like sending her children to college. She was still smarting from the fact that her mother was too cheap to send her. But this is not to say that Rita was comfortable paying for college. She limited the amount of tuition she would pay and insisted that her children attend local, less expensive colleges no matter how well they had done in high school. Gary learned from his parents that having a good time was important; he even admitted that he was somewhat jealous of his parents' ability to do so. But Gary also saw his father's lifestyle as somewhat irresponsible, and he too feared he would end up with little. With Rita, Gary felt safe and secure, but paralyzed.

No wonder this couple had ferocious control struggles over money. Gary was a little too loose with money and Rita was too tight. Just as other couples do when stuck, they insist that the therapist be the judge and jury. Who is right and who is wrong? I pointed out that my opinion about how the couple treat their finances should be of no consequence. The issue in question is whether they can negotiate a satisfactory compromise. I could see both points of view: Rita was so cautious about spending money that she led an austere existence. And because of her distrust of financial professionals, she did not protect herself from inflation and heavy taxes. One could say that her need for control was eventually going to cause her to lose control (and money). Gary, while not the spendthrift his wife made him out to be, was not saving enough to enjoy a comfortable retirement. Like his father, he lived in the moment.

As mentioned, receiving conflicting messages about control from the family of origin is not the only way to develop a conflict about control. Let us now look at the second major source of this type of conflict: trauma.

Trauma

According to van der Kolk (2014): "Trauma happens to us, our friends, our families, and our neighbors" (p. 1). He referred to it as "a much larger public health issue, arguably the greatest threat to our national well-being" (p. 350). Approximately 70% of adults in the United States experience at least one traumatic event in their lifetime (Sidran Institute, 2018). And you do not have to experience the trauma directly; if those around you are impacted, you may end up collateral damage (van der Kolk, 2014).

People who have been re-exposed to the same or similar trauma often experience intense or unwanted physical and emotional reactions—many have panic attacks (SingleCare, 2021). These feelings may come on rapidly or be delayed. The clinical term used to describe this experience is widely known as post-traumatic stress disorder (PTSD). Approximately 5% or more than 13 million people in the United States have PTSD at any given time (Sidran Institute, 2018). van der Kolk and McFarlane (1996) wrote:

> The critical element that makes an event traumatic is the subjective assessment by victims of how threatened and helpless they feel. So, although the reality of extraordinary events are at the core of PTSD, the meaning that the victims attach to these events are as fundamental as the trauma itself.
>
> (p. 6)

Neuroscience has helped us to understand how life experiences can change the structure and function of the brain, and especially how trauma can change our brain's development. As a result, scientists and mental health clinicians have been better able to help the traumatized gain control over deleterious reactions to stress (Porges, 2011; van der Kolk, 2014). People who have been traumatized try hard to maintain control in their lives to avoid re-traumatization. This may include control over their experiences, their bodies, and especially those closest to them. Because this takes a huge amount of energy, they often pay a hefty price both emotionally and physically, and control struggles are inevitable.

Pre-Conflict Trauma

A conflict about control can be "caused" by a traumatic life event if experienced young enough—or before the individual's internal conflict has been internalized—such as early childhood sexual abuse or the loss of a parent.

Kathy lost her father when she was four years old. He left home one day for work and never returned—he was killed in a plane crash. Kathy's mother and sisters never discussed the issue. A funeral was held and not a word was ever spoken. Kathy married three times and each time she found reasons to terminate the relationship. Kathy's mother was overwhelmed caring for three daughters on her own. She managed to hold a full-time job, but she did not have enough energy left to structure her family. As a result, her daughters did as they pleased. Kathy married a fourth time to her current husband Jack.

Jack came from a close-knit, highly structured home life. Like his father, he was very studious and eventually became a history professor. Jack instantly fell for Kathy's beauty and vivaciousness. Unlike him, he saw her as "full-of-life." What he missed, however, was Kathy's need to control the couple's distance. Not used to so much space, Jack began to demand more of Kathy, but she rebelled. She insisted on separate bedrooms and even requested her own part-time apartment. This behavior was foreign to Jack's world, but he gave in to keep Kathy from leaving him. Ironically, Kathy never requested a divorce; she simply wanted control over the distance in the relationship. She decided if, and when the couple would sleep in the same room, have sex, and socialize together. She wanted to stay together at a distance she could tolerate. In treatment, Jack revealed that Kathy treats all her friends and siblings in the same manner: they are connected, but she controls the space between.

Esther's experience is another good example of the impact early trauma can have on conflict. Esther was a young child when she was a prisoner in Auschwitz. Having lost her parents in the concentration camps she somehow managed to survive and was eventually transported to relatives in the United States. She met her husband Saul at a Jewish function, and they hit it off. They had much in common since he too was a camp survivor. Although Saul seemed to adapt to his new and much safer environment, Esther grew to be angry, distrusting, and controlling. She was fighting with Saul as well as her daughter and son-in-law. Her need to control them all put enormous pressure on the family. It was so bad, Saul worried that his children would soon disown he and Esther to save their marriages.

Esther was stubbornly guarded in treatment. She refused to open-up and acted as if she were being interrogated. When I offered an intervention, she would usually roll her eyes or grunt disapprovingly. She clearly did not trust me and gave the impression that she felt I had no idea what I was doing. When I asked why she felt the need to challenge her husband and children, she said that somebody had to look after them. When I challenged her on her need to control the treatment, she pulled her glasses down to the tip of her nose, looked out of the top of them and said that she was finished being controlled by others. It did not work out the last time—meaning the Holocaust.

Post-Conflict Trauma

If the trauma occurs after the conflict has been internalized—as in the case of juvenile or adult sexual abuse, physical assault, life-threatening illness, a major loss, a contemptuous divorce, or war—the trauma can serve to "reinforce" the conflict.

Michael and Melissa were a couple in their early 40s. By Michael's standards, his wife Melissa was a bright, beautiful woman. The couple first met in college and from Michael's perspective it was love at first sight. Michael immediately pushed for a commitment from Melissa, and she acquiesced. But Michael proved too much for his wife: He was increasingly controlling and jealous, putting her down to contain her and to increase her dependence upon him. He even insisted she not work. While Melissa's parents were divorced and her father estranged from the family, Michael was catered to as an only child. He claimed that his parents were caring but they were both controlling and intrusive.

Initially Melissa enjoyed the security Michael provided, but soon tired of it and left him for another man. Michael was devastated—he even needed to be hospitalized. While Michael admitted he was controlling, this trauma served to increase rather than decrease his need for control. He avoided relationships for several years, and when he resumed, he went out with women who he considered far beneath him. He vowed never to let his guard down with a woman again. When Michael finally decided to commit to a woman—Beth—he developed a severe alcohol problem, a method he unconsciously employed to avoid giving himself completely to her. Losing his wife did not loosen Michael's conflict, it exacerbated it.

References

Bowen, M. (1978). *Family therapy in clinical practice*. Aronson.

Boszormenyi-Nagy, I., & Spark, G. (1973). *Invisible loyalties*. Harper & Row.

Kleber, R. (2019). Trauma and public mental health: A focused review. *Frontiers in Psychiatry*, *10*, 1–6. https://doi.org/10.3389//psyt.2019.00451

Porges, S. (2011). *The polyvagal theory: Neurophysiological foundations of emotions, attachment, communication, and self-regulation*. Norton.

Sidran Institute (2018, December 10). *Traumatic stress disorder fact sheet*. https://www.sidran.org/wp-content/uploads/2018/11/Post-Traumatic-Stress-Disorder-Fact-Sheet-.pdf

Singlecare (2021, January 21). *PTSD statistics 2021*. Checkup. www.singlecare.com/blog/news/ptsd-statistics/

Tannen, D. (2011). *That is not what I meant: How conversational style makes or breaks relationships*. Harper.

Toman, W. (1976). *Family constellation: Its effects on personality and social behavior*. Springer.

van der Kolk, B.A. (2014). *The body keeps the score: Brain, mind, and body in the healing of trauma*. Penguin.

van der Kolk, B.A., & McFarlane, A.C. (1996). The black hole of trauma. In B.A. van der Kolk, A.C. McFarlane, & L. Weisaeth (Eds.), *Traumatic stress: The effects of overwhelming experience on mind, body, and society* (pp. 3–23). Guilford.

3   The Unconscious Process of Mate Selection

Mate preference is important to consider in the future of a couple's ability to avoid or resolve control struggles. It is hard enough for one partner to change, but when that partner's dysfunction is supported by their mate, it can be an impossible task. I am frequently asked: What is the major cause of divorce? And I always answer: "Marriage." Who we pick often determines the fate of our relationship.

Mate Choice

Couples who are having difficulty often conclude that they are "a bad match," and that their struggles over certain relational issues are an indication of this. But this is usually code for they do not understand or wish to know the true cause of their struggle. A female client told me she decided not to attend couples therapy to help her husband work on his low sexual drive. It was her belief that he should not have had this issue in the first place. "Sex between two people is natural, especially a husband and wife," she said. "If we are having a problem, it means we should not be together. Being married should not be hard."

The client was making two distinct but related points: First, she implied that a good relationship should come naturally. And second, she suggested that if there is a problem in a relationship it signifies that the relationship was not meant to be. But she was wrong on both counts. Relationships are a challenge that require consistent work and perseverance. For most, cultivating a healthy, intimate relationship is one of life's biggest feats. And in all my years of treating couples, I have never seen a bad match. I have seen destructive matches in which people abuse or betray one another, but from a theoretical perspective I would still not consider these mismatches. A colleague commented: "If one partner has had a low sex drive for many years, it is most likely that the other partner does not need sex that badly." The implication here is that people choose each other out of mutual collusion.

Darwin (1871/2004) brought the concept of mate selection in humans to the world in his book, *The Descent of Man*. Elaborating on "sexual selection"—a vehicle for "natural selection"—he wrote that humans too, adapt and survive with the help of sexual choice and reproduction. Darwin generally believed that

DOI: 10.4324/9781003159100-4

animals and humans could choose who to mate with—something we humans demonstrate everyday by consciously choosing our mates based on income and education (Fales & Fisher, 2016), physical attraction (Fugère et al., 2017), physical proximity (Jonason et al., 2017), individual and dyadic reciprocity of attraction (Back et al., 2011), and similarity of interests (Byrne, 1971).

Biological factors have also been found to play a part in mate selection. Fisher et al. (2007) claimed that romantic love is one of three brain systems that evolved to direct reproduction: Sex drive evolved to encourage individuals to have sex with others; attraction evolved to pursue a specific person; and attachment evolved to motivate people to stay together. The authors claimed that activities of central oxytocin (a peptide hormone and neuropeptide), which plays a role in social bonding, reproduction, and childbirth, and vasopressin (a diuretic hormone), have all been associated with partner preference and attachment; the dopaminergic pathways in the brain are associated specifically with partner preference.

While all these factors have proved valuable in understanding mate selection, this book is primarily concerned with the "unconscious psychological" process that steers long-term mate choice. And there is much to support this phenomenon in the professional literature.

Psychoanalysis

Jung (1931/1954) believed in the strong, unconscious influence our parents have on our choice of mates. In his paper "Marriage as a Psychological Relationship" he wrote:

> The relationship of the young man to his mother, and of the girl to her father is the determining factor in this respect. It is the strength of the bond to the parents that unconsciously influences the choice of husband or wife, either positively or negatively.
>
> (pp. 190–191)

And Freud (1905/1953), ever the determinist, also believed that we choose people who remind us of our opposite-sex parents. In *Three Essays on the Theory of Sexuality*, he wrote:

> It often happens that a young man falls in love seriously for the first time with a mature woman, or a girl with an elderly man in a position of authority; this is, clearly an echo of the phase of development that we have been discussing, since these figures can re-animate pictures of their mother or father. There can be no doubt that every object-choice whatever is based, though less closely, on these prototypes.
>
> (p. 228)

While many studies have generally supported psychoanalytic theory (Geher, 2000; Jedlicka, 1980, 1984), there are some interesting divergencies. Heffernan et al. (2018) found that biracial people chose mates that resembled their parents, but that the sex of the person was inconsequential. Specifically, individuals did not significantly choose someone of the same race as the opposite-sex parent. And Perrett (2017) found men and women favor those that reminded them of their opposite-sex parent based primarily on facial recognition. The author believed that people are attracted to those we are most familiar with and can therefore better identify with, including their own countrymen.

Object Relations Therapy

Dicks (1967/1993) adapted Fairbairn's (1952/1990) Object Relations model to work with couples. Dicks contended that while we consciously choose our mates based on general compatibility and sexual attraction, our unconscious plays a big role in mate selection. He claimed that the unconscious mind seeks out complementarity in a potential mate based on childhood experience with our primary caregivers, usually our mothers.

Basic object relations theory posits that as infants we are wholly dependent on the primary caregiver and therefore cannot tolerate perceiving her in a negative light. To defend against the reality that she holds both good (loving) and bad (rejecting) aspects, we internalize and repress these aspects, and split our central ego or self into two ego subtypes: the exciting object (to protect the illusion that the mother is all good we make ourselves bad) and the rejecting object (to protect against the pain of a dismissive mother we idealize her good aspects thus creating a good object for ourselves).

According to Dicks (1967/1993), we look to potential mates to help us re-find these "lost aspects" of ourselves and in turn, to complete us. A healthy marriage or relationship allows for the de-repression of these lost parts via one's partner—it specifically allows for insight, empowerment, and acceptance of our true selves, and the entire range of aspects that make us human. Scharff and Scharff (1997) found that an unhealthy relationship serves to reinforce previous repression, maladaptive defenses, and a dysfunctional fit. Most couples are not conscious of their fit until something disturbs it, thereby exposing repressed parts of unconscious needs and expectations that are unmet.

To explain the unconscious communication and dynamics between mates, Dicks (1967/1993) incorporated the concept introduced by Melanie Klein (1946)—*projective identification*—or the defense mechanism one uses to project qualities unacceptable to the self onto another person. Dicks offered the following:

> This joint personality or integrate enabled each half to rediscover lost aspects of their primary object relations, which they split off or repressed, and which

they were, in their involvement with the spouse, re-experiencing by projective identification. The sense of belonging can be understood on the hypothesis that at a deeper level there are perceptions of the partner and consequent attitudes towards him or her *as if* the other was part of oneself was valued: spoilt and cherished, or denigrated and persecuted.

(p. 69)

Attachment Theory

Bowlby (1969, 1973, 1980) studied the reliance of infants and young children on their primary caregiver—the mother—and the distress they experience when separated from her. Bowlby believed we have two complementary internal models: (1) a model of the self that reflects how loveable we are in the eyes of our attachment figure; and (2) a model of the other which concerns how responsive our attachment figure is perceived. As a child we look to the caregiver's consistent empathic responses for comfort and support. If this occurs, our worthiness is reinforced, and we internalize a secure attachment style. If the caregiver has been inconsistent, our attachment to the caregiver will be insecure and lead to insecure attachment capability. These internal attachment models follow us as children into adulthood and can have a profound impact on our romantic relationships (Hazan & Shaver, 1987).

Extending Bowlby's work, Ainsworth et al. (1978), have delineated three attachment styles in response to an infant's expectations of the primary caregiver: *secure, anxious/ambivalent,* and the *avoidant.* The authors claimed that differences in infant attachment styles are among the determinants of adult romantic attachment styles. The secure adult is characterized by trust and positivity; the anxious/ambivalent type struggles mightily with joining in an intimate relationship which often proves to be simultaneously exciting and excruciating—sometimes bordering on obsessive; and the avoidant adult demonstrates a lack of trust and a fear of closeness.

In their classic article, "Romantic Love Conceptualized as an Attachment Process," Hazan and Shaver (1987) supported these traits and tendencies. They wrote the following: "secure respondents characterized their love experiences as friendly, happy, and trusting, whereas avoidant subjects reported fear of closeness, and anxious/ambivalent subjects described relationships marked by jealously, emotional highs and lows, and desire for reciprocation" (p. 518).

Considering Hazan and Shaver's (1987) preference for the 3-classification system (*secure, anxious/ambivalent,* and *avoidant*), and Bartholomew and Horowitz's (1991) 4-style classification (*secure, preoccupied, dismissing-avoidant, fearful-avoidant*), Holmes and Johnson (2009) compiled a study of the literature on adult attachment and romantic partner preference. Three hypotheses have emerged from these studies: (1) individuals prefer partners with a *similar* attachment style: avoidant individuals will show preference for an avoidant person or an anxious person will seek out an anxious partner; (2) those with a *complementary* attachment style prefer partners who will confirm attachment-related expectations: anxious individuals prefer avoidant individuals and *vice versa*, confirming the anxious partner's expectations of others to distance, and the avoidant partner's expectations of others to cling; and (3) individuals with a secure attachment style provides *attachment security*, which is preferred by all individuals regardless of attachment style. These individuals make security a priority and seek out secure individuals; anxious individuals are a second choice followed by avoidant ones.

The findings of their extensive review suggested that when given a choice of hypothetical partners (someone they could be attracted to), individuals based their partner preference on similarity and attachment-security. For example, an anxious partner was attracted to either a secure or similarly anxious partner, and an avoidant partner was attracted to a secure or similarly avoidant partner based on a shared need for distance and autonomy. For long-term relationships, individuals demonstrated a preference for a complementary partner. For example, an anxious individual might prefer the complementary avoidant partner and *vice versa*.

More than any other model of psychotherapy, attachment theory has caught the attention of both the professional and lay audiences. This is thanks primarily to the work of Susan Johnson (2019, 2008), who applied the attachment theory to working with couples in her model: Emotionally Focused Therapy (EFS).

Systems Therapy

Some systems therapists also take a deterministic view on mate selection. Bowen (1978), for example, believed people who select one another have similar levels of emotional autonomy from their respective families of origin. His concept of *differentiation of self* is defined as the degree to which one can balance emotional and intellectual functioning, and intimacy and autonomy in relationships.

There are two aspects of differentiation: (1) intrapsychic differentiation: being able to regulate our thoughts and feelings—poorly differentiated people are more emotionally reactive; and (2) interpersonal differentiation: the capacity to separate our experiences from those we are connected to—the degree to which we can allow ourselves to become intimately involved with someone but not lose our self in the process. Bowen believed that a healthy balance between closeness and autonomy allows for a more intimate connection between partners and fosters relationship growth.

And Whitaker (1974) contended that the necessity for completing oneself by mating is an underlying driving force. Choosing a mate is mostly an unconscious way to fulfill a need to return to one's family of origin without having to go back there. The developer of the Symbolic-experiential approach to treatment, Whitaker supported Bowen's belief that therapy should stimulate the growth of the individual alongside the growth of the system.

Master Conflict Therapy

When it comes to partner preference, MCT is also unconscious and deterministic. Partners are destined to choose someone with the "same" internal conflict, and they do so with uncanny accuracy. I have asserted before that if you enter a room full of people with the intention of finding a mate—no matter how many people are present—you will inevitably choose someone with the same master conflict (Betchen, 2010).

How this matching process occurs is almost hypnotic in nature, with each partner often missing anything about the other that may warn of potential trouble. I first witnessed this when as a 20-something, I was to meet my best friend at the time, Jerry, at a local bar/restaurant. When I arrived, I found Jerry with another young man who I will refer to as Keith. Keith was a handsome, articulate guy who I soon realized was a misogynist.

Keith was rude to every woman we tried to talk to that night, but I assumed that because of his good looks no one reacted negatively to his provoking antics. To my surprise, a woman I will call Jill, seemed rather smitten with him. When it was clear that Jill was interested, both Keith and Jerry invited her to have dinner with us. Naïvely, I went along thinking that Keith would settle down, but instead the dynamic deteriorated. After criticizing her physical appearance, Keith used graphic sex to express what he would like to do to Jill. He seemed to be trying hard to be as disrespectful to her as he could.

I kept my head down and tried to focus on my dinner without becoming nauseous. My plan was to eat and leave. Suddenly, however, Jill gave me an opening. She turned to me and asked: "Why are you so quiet?" Without hesitation I sarcastically responded: "I am too busy listening to you being abused." With that, one of the boys kicked me under the table as if to say you are ruining our fun. But I persisted. I wanted to save Jill from the world of pain which would inevitably follow.

Jill did seem intrigued with my use of the term "abuse." She reacted as if I handed her the results of a complex research experiment, or the secret sauce to grandmother's pizza. I thought . . . maybe she will get it and leave, or at least give Keith a good reprimanding. But she stayed on and the look in her eyes when she gazed at Keith told me that all hope was lost; Jill was madly in love.

Near the end of dinner Jill had somewhere to be and proudly handed Keith her telephone number. She even promised him that he would enjoy her body if he followed up on her invitation. To me, it appeared Jill felt the need to take a few more punches before she could allow herself to be treated better by a man. It was at that point that I knew Jill and Keith were made for each other. Jill had found her prince.

Unfortunately, many people refuse to believe they have little control over such an important and intimate decision. This denial makes perfect sense from a psychological and theoretical point of view. For example, if two people accept full responsibility for choosing one another, they then must take equal responsibility if anything goes wrong in the relationship. After all, they chose each other.

Nevertheless, it is infinitely easier to separate yourself from your partner, as if they have a problem completely independent of you. It also allows unconscious conflicts to seamlessly join.

Mate selection from the MCT perspective does not always apply to one-night stands. It can, but it usually pertains to long-term relationships or marriage. Behind the choice for a mate is the need for a couple to collude in the preservation of their master conflict—a tricky proposition given that one partner usually disagrees with the other, giving off the impression that the couple are "different." However, they are quite similar in the most important way—they share the same conflict. MCT contends that it is not the differences in couples that can tear them apart, but their unconscious "similarity." Unfortunately, the couples therapist must contend with "two" people who are staunchly supporting the maintenance of their "shared" conflict. I refer to such couples as "twins-in-conflict" (Betchen, 2010; Betchen & Davidson, 2018).

This is also relevant to long-term extramarital affairs. An affair, perhaps over any other relational dynamic, generates a hypnotic attraction to a lover. Much of this attraction, however, is external and therefore mistakenly perceived by the cheater to be much different than attraction to the primary partner. Lovers are often described as affectionate, caring, empathic, and sexually willing—the opposite perception of the primary partner. But under analysis, the lover and mate are similar in conflict. Because it takes time, and often professional help to reveal conflict similarity—in combination with the unfaithful partner's denial—the unfaithful partner rarely figures this out until the affair has taken hold. In the end, however, the unfaithful mate discovers what the master conflict theorist already knows: that the unfaithful partner has chosen his primary partner again, albeit in a different form.

Consider the complex case of Colleen and Brad. The couple was in therapy primarily because of Colleen's open affair. Brad claimed that he wanted his wife to end this relationship so that he and Colleen could work on their marriage, but Colleen refused. Feeling stuck, the couple's therapist referred Colleen to me for individual therapy to see if I could help her break free of her lover. In the following exchange Colleen realizes that her lover and husband are one in the same in a most important way:

Therapist: Colleen, what is so appealing about your lover?

Colleen: He always compliments me, and he wants to make love to me all the time. We can talk about intimate things and he always has his arm around me and caresses me.

Therapist: What's your husband like?

Colleen: He's a narcissist. He's cheap, he hides things from me, and he rarely has time for me. He's more interested in getting together with his friends than with me.

Therapist: Is your lover married?

Colleen: Yes.

Therapist: How long has he been married?

Colleen: About 25 years.

Therapist: That's a long time. I assume he is unhappy in his marriage.

Colleen: Yes, he and his wife haven't even slept together for years. He says she's more focused on her career than on him. It seems his wife and my husband are similar.

Therapist: I hear your husband hates couples therapy. Is that true?

Colleen: Yeah, he thinks it's a waste of time. He's always giving the couples therapist a hard time.

Therapist: So, he doesn't really want to fix this situation?

Colleen: I never thought of it that way. He thinks I should just stop the affair, and all will be well. He doesn't really know how to fix anything.

Therapist: Has your lover been to couples therapy with his wife?

Colleen: No, he doesn't believe in it either. He says I'm his therapist.

Therapist: So, your lover and husband are the same person, but one is taller than the other.

Colleen: No . . . wait. What do you mean?

Therapist: Well, if you and your lover run off together and experience some relationship difficulty—which is inevitable—he too, might not want to fix it, or have no clue how. He might not even want to. It sounds as if he is a fair-weather lover.

Colleen: That's hard to believe.

Therapist: Well, has he ever told you that he's leaving his wife for you?

Colleen: No.

Therapist: So, he has no plans to leave his wife or to work on his marriage. It seems he is strangely content to let things brew without a solution. Doesn't this remind you of someone?

Colleen: I never looked at it this way. Maybe I'll pursue this with him.

Therapist: You mean like a test of some sort.

Colleen: Yes.

Colleen did pursue her lover about his desire to problem-solve and found that he was like her husband in this area. Not instantly, but soon she ended both her affair and her marriage.

The unconscious replication of choosing a mate with the same internal conflict is one of the reasons why the divorce rates for second and third marriages are so high: The divorce rates for first marriages is approximately 50%; the rate for second marriages is about 60%, and the rate for third marriages is 73% (World Population Review, 2021). With limited insight, individuals are more likely to replicate their failures. Even those who have an affair and marry experience a 75% divorce rate (Divorcesource.com, 2017). When people use the term "love at first sight," it might be more accurate to refer to it as "conflict at first sight."

As mentioned in "Chapter 1. Introduction: Control and Conflict," all people have internal conflicts but only one dominates: the master conflict. Although several other master conflicts have been identified, this book is focused on only one—the one that is all too common and particularly troublesome to a couple: *control versus out-of-control*. Individuals with this conflict choose one another to mate with and in turn, create a formidable internal bond in which each partner experiences being in and out-of-control. When neither partner is too in control or too out-of-control, the couple and their conflict is said to be balanced and few if any relational symptoms should appear.

To maintain the integrity of the conflict, partners regulate themselves and each other by consistently shifting slightly from one side of the conflict to the other. If the conflict becomes unbalanced, the couple will experience serious, long-lasting control struggles until it is rebalanced. Control struggles can operate in a variety of relational contexts: finances, parenting, and sex, to name a few.

References

Ainsworth, M.D.S., Blehar, M.C., Waters, E., & Wall, S. (1978). *Patterns of attachment: Assessed in the strange situation and at home*. Erlbaum.

Back, M., Penke, L., Schmukle, S.C., Sachse, K., Borkenau, P., & Asendorpf, J.B. (2011). Why mate choices are not as reciprocal as we assume: The role of personality, flirting, and physical attractiveness. *European Journal of Personality*, *25*, 120–132. https://doi.org/10.1002/per.806

Bartholomew, K., & Horowitz, L.M. (1991). Attachment styles among young adults: A test of a four-category model. *Journal of Personality and Social Psychology*, *61*, 226–244. https://doi.org/10.1037/0022-3514.61.2.226

Betchen, S. (2010). *Magnetic partners: Discover how the hidden conflict that once attracted you to each other is now driving you apart*. Free Press.

Betchen, S., & Davidson, H. (2018). *Master conflict therapy: A new model for practicing couples and sex therapy*. Routledge.

Bowen, M. (1978). *Family therapy in clinical practice*. Aronson.

Bowlby, J. (1969). *Attachment and loss: Vol. 1. Attachment*. Basic Books.

Bowlby, J. (1973). *Attachment and loss: Vol. 2. Separation: Anxiety and anger*. Basic Books.

Bowlby, J. (1980). *Attachment and loss: Vol. 3. Loss: Sadness and depression*. Basic Books.

Byrne, D. (1971). *The attraction paradigm*. Academic Press.

Darwin, C. (1871/2004). *The descent of man*. Penguin Classics.

Dicks, H.V. (1967/1993). *Marital tensions: Clinical studies towards a psychological theory of interaction*. Karnac.

Divorcesource.com (2017, February 15). *When marriages begin as affairs*. www.divorcesource.com/blog/when-marriages-begin-as-affairs/

Fairbairn, W.R.D. (1952/1990). *Psychoanalytic study of the personality*. Routledge.

Fales, M., & Fisher, F. (2016). Mating markets and bargaining hands: Mate preferences for attractiveness and resources in two national U.S. studies. *Personality and Individual Differences, 88,* 78–87. https://doi.org/10.1016/j.paid.2015.08.041

Fisher, H., Aron, A., & Brown, L. (December 2007). Romantic love: A mammalian brain system for mate choice. *Philosophical Transactions of the Royal Society B: Biological Sciences, 361,* 2173–2186. https://doi.org/10/1098/rstb.2006.1938

Freud, S. (1905/1953). A case of hysteria, three essays on sexuality and other works. In J. Strachey (Ed. and Trans.), *The standard edition of the complete psychological works of Sigmund Freud* (Vol. 7, pp. 135–200). Hogarth Press and the Institute for Psychoanalysis.

Fugère, M.A., Chabot, C., Doucette, K., & Cousins, A. (2017). The importance of physical attractiveness to the mate choices of women and their mothers. *Evolutionary Psychological Science, 3,* 243–252. https://doi.org/10.1007/s40806-017-0092-x

Geher, G. (2000). Perceived and actual characteristics of parents and partners: A test of a Freudian model of mate selection. *Current Psychology, 19,* 194–214. https://doi.org/10.1007/s12144-000-1015-7

Hazan, C., & Shaver, P. (1987). Romantic love conceptualized as an attachment process. *Journal of Personality and Social Psychology, 52,* 511–524. https://doi.org/10.1037/0022-3514/87/500.75

Heffernan, M., Chong, J., & Fraley, C. (2018). Are people attracted to others who resemble their opposite-sex parents? An examination of mate preferences and parental ethnicity among biracial individuals. *Social Psychological and Personality Science, 10,* 856–863. https://doi.org/10/1177/1948550618794679

Holmes, B., & Johnson, K. (2009). Adult attachment and romantic partner preference: A review. *Journal of Social and Personality Psychology, 26,* 833–852. https://doi.org/10.1177/0265407509345653

Jedlicka, D. (1980). A test of the psychoanalytic theory of mate selection. *Journal of Social Psychology, 112,* 295–299. https://doi.org/10.1080/00224545.1980.9924331

Jedlicka, D. (1984). Indirect parental influence on mate choice: A test of the psychoanalytic theory. *Journal of Marriage and Family, 46,* 65–70. https://doi.org/10.2307/351864

Johnson, S. (2008). *Hold me tight: Seven conversations for a lifetime of love.* Little, Brown Spark.

Johnson, S. (2019). *The practice of emotionally focused marital therapy: Creating connection* (3rd ed.). Routledge.

Jonason, P.K., Nolland, M., & Tyler, M.D. (2017). Incorporating geographic distance into mate preference research: Necessities and luxuries. *Personal Relationships, 24,* 471–473. https://doi.org/10.1111/pere.12199

Jung, C.G. (1931/1954). The development of personality: Papers on child psychology, education, and related subjects. Marriage as a psychological relationship. In R.F.C. Hull (Trans.), *The collected works of C.G. Jung* (Vol. 17, pp. 187–201). Princeton University Press.

Klein, M. (1946). Notes on some schizoid mechanisms. *The Psychoanalytic Quarterly, 18,* 122–132. https://doi.org/10.1080/21674086.1949.11925749

Perrett, D. (2017). *In your face: The new science of human attraction.* Palgrave-McMillan.

Scharff, D., & Scharff, J. (1997). Object relations couple therapy. *American Journal of Psychotherapy, 51,* 141–173. https://doi.org/10.1176/appi.psychotherapy.1997.512.141

Whitaker, C. (1974). Marriage: Before, during and after. *Family Court Review, 12,* 6. https://doi.org/10.1111/j.174.tb01204x

World Population Review (2021). *Divorce rate by state 2021.* Retrieved July 28, 2021, from https://worldpopulationreview.com/state-rankings/divorce-rate-by-state

4   Controlling Styles

Partners who find themselves locked in control struggles demonstrate one of two predominantly different styles of control: (1) they try to control their significant other; or (2) they try to maintain control by refusing to allow their significant other to control them. Some partners exhibit both styles, but this is highly dependent on context. For example, a male client overtly controlled the finances in his marriage but consistently avoided having to perform any domestic chores assigned by his wife.

Ironically, for those couples who have an unbalanced, internal control conflict, neither style may provide long-lasting control. Two partners with the same style, for example, may join to form a *symmetrical* dynamic; because of their similarity they may seem like a perfect fit. But because they use the same tactics when battling for control, they are prone to volatility. It is much more likely, however, that partners with different styles will match up in the hopes of complementing each other, and this is what the couples therapist will encounter most often. This *complementary* union may appear, especially on the surface, to be a more harmonious fit. Each partner may stir interest by bringing something new and different to the relationship, and they may also use different control tactics that might not directly clash as much as similar tactics would. Nevertheless, their differences can create confusion and misunderstanding.

Those partners that try to exert too much control often provoke avoidance and in turn experience less control. Those who try to avoid being controlled use techniques that often make things worse; they tend to inadvertently provoke their significant others to increase control. It is no wonder that couples with internal conflicts about control easily end up in control struggles. The following sections address the ways in which partners attempt to control and to avoid control. Some of these tactics are applied consciously and others unconsciously. Notice how counterproductive they can be.

DOI: 10.4324/9781003159100-5

Techniques Used to Control

Verbal Threats

There are several different ways to attempt to verbally control your partner and one of the most common is to use verbal threats (Brogaard, 2015). Verbal threats exist on a continuum with a mild threat on one end and a threat to physically harm on the other. There seems to be a correlation between the degree one feels the need for control and the seriousness of the threat used to gain or regain control. The purpose of a mild threat might be to warn your partner that you may no longer perform some household duty or something that your partner values. For example, a female client threatened never to get a dog unless her husband agreed to contribute to its care. Another example was that of a male client who threatened to withhold money to secure control over family finances.

A more serious threat, however, might be to warn that you are considering having an affair or a separation. Some partners have gone as far as to hire a lawyer as a threat to gain control in the relationship even though they had no real intention of divorcing. A former female client consistently threatened her meek husband with divorce whenever he expressed some displeasure with her. She even hired a lawyer to send him a letter threatening divorce. The husband told me that although he did not appreciate his wife's control, he was too afraid to challenge her for fear that she might leave. But he soon began to exhibit episodic temper tantrums over unrelated and innocuous events which proved to be symptomatic of his displeasure.

Verbally threatening your mate in public is sometimes effective in gaining temporary control, but the humiliating effect it may have can cause serious relationship problems. For example, a female client told me that her husband was not very social and that his anxiety level would go up when surrounded by people in social situations. Wary not to incite him, the wife almost never held parties at their house. However, she eventually reached her threshold of tolerance when she was prohibited from having one or two friends over; this too, would anger her husband.

> When my friends visit, my husband finds something to complain about like we were too loud, or we disturbed his nap. Then he would scream at me in front of my friends and even insult them. He asked one friend if she were here because she had no other place to go. I really cannot take this any longer. I feel like a prisoner in my own home.

Threatening your partner with physical harm is the scariest attempt at verbal control. One spouse threatens to hit the other to gain control. Some even raise their fists or pull a weapon. While some of this is posturing, it must be taken seriously by all those involved. Physical harm will be dealt with in a latter section, but it usually ends badly for all parties.

Regardless of the specific threat, partners use whatever they believe will most startle their counterparts and afford them greater control. Partners know how to scare their mates; they know each other's weaknesses. To attempt to ensure control over the other, some partners use tactics that do not merit the gravity of the situation. I refer to this as the need to "bring a gun to a knife fight."

A very anxious male client was raised by parents who grew up poor. From this experience, he learned to be very conservative with money to the point of living a life of deprivation. Pleasure and comfort were considered luxuries. Unhappy with his wife's spending habits, he destroyed her credit card when it reached a balance of $500. He then threatened to leave her unless she curbed her ways. The wife understood her husband's position but felt that he was overreacting and needed help. But because she took his threat seriously, she acquiesced and adapted to his lifestyle. She said that being controlled was cheaper than a divorce, but time demonstrated that she could not live under his yoke.

Blaming

Gottman and Silver (2015) said it is okay to complain but not to blame; sound wisdom. But too often couples use "blame" as a technique to try and gain control in a relationship. The adage "the best defense is a good offense" applies here. If you are constantly verbally attacking your mate, there is little opportunity for your partner to counterattack. I have seen this technique used more often by women than men. Young females have been historically discouraged from being physically aggressive—it was considered unladylike. Rather, they were taught to hide negative feelings and to settle their disagreements in a verbal, civilized manner; some unfortunately, were trained to be passive aggressive. Men, however, were encouraged to protect their masculinity and settle matters even if it meant physical confrontation—which it often did. While women are becoming more assertive and men less violent, there is still enough difference in the way the two genders communicate to cause relationship difficulty.

Some individuals use the blaming technique even after the other partner has accepted blame. It is as if the accusing partner wishes to make sure their counterpart remains in a submissive position. A female client complained that her husband never initiated conversation, or sex. The husband expressed remorse and said that his behavior was related to an abusive childhood. He further explained that he always tried to get by in life by hiding—a technique he learned growing up with violent parents. He admitted that he was scared but expressed a willingness to work to be more present in his marriage. Rather than express appreciation or empathy, his wife complained even louder about her husband's insufficiencies and continued to do so for the rest of the session. By all accounts she should have been pleased to gain some control in her marriage, but she wanted more. Eventually the husband began to realize that he could never give her enough control and the relationship deteriorated.

Emotional Manipulation (Crying)

Crying may be a legitimate sign of anxiety, depression, grief, or a way to dilute anger (Zoppi, 2020; Wise, 2020; Wong, 2019). According to Wong (2019), it may also be gender-based because women have been historically raised to suppress their anger. But crying can also be used as a tool to try and gain control. Crying is effective because it can be paradoxical. The crier appears vulnerable, and is usually perceived as nonthreatening: a weak, victimized individual. But what may appear on the outside might not represent the underlying objective: disarming control.

When we do not feel attacked, it is hard to strike. I am sure you have heard: "Never kick someone when they are down." The partner who is quick to cry, often stops the other from continuing to hold them responsible. Even when enraged with a partner if he/she begins to cry our natural concern creeps in and at best, we become confused. A man broke down and sobbed uncontrollably after his wife had discovered his affair. The wife then commented to me: "I don't know whether to kill him or feel sorry for him." But she did remain ambivalent towards him.

A husband reported to me that he was no longer interested in having sex with his wife. After obtaining a history of his relationship, I hypothesized that he was angry with her for forcing him to suppress his feelings, especially his anger. For some time, the man did not believe me, but I encouraged him to test my concept out. On a double date the man observed that his wife paid far more attention to her friend's husband than to him. Later that evening he gently approached her about this, and she instantly began to cry. The man reported to me that his complaint was rather mild but that his wife was still able to evoke guilt in him and so he apologized to her. In treatment the man got in touch with his anger and his wife's manipulation, much of which was unconscious. Once he confronted her, although she cried, he paid no attention and stood his ground. As his wife got used to being confronted, the man's sex drive returned. His feelings were no longer suppressed, and his wife curbed her crying response.

Physical Abuse (Bullying and Stalking)

Physically intimidating, stalking, restraining, or striking is used far too often to try and control a mate's behavior. According to the Center for Disease Control and Prevention (2021), domestic violence effects 10 million people in the United States every year. More than one in five women and more than one in seven men report having experienced rape, physical violence, or stalking by an intimate partner in their lifetime. Accordingly, 85% of domestic violence victims are female and 15% are male.

A female client reported that whenever she voiced an opinion that her husband did not agree with, he would push her against a wall and put one hand on her throat while holding her with the other. This was to stop her from talking. Another woman claimed that when her husband wanted to dominate her, he would lean over her and put his face close to hers while telling her to shut up. She said it was terrifying. After some counseling, she finally threatened to leave him if he ever did this again. And while he acquiesced, she held it against him for years.

A male client reported that he wanted to stop seeing a woman he had dated for two weeks, but she would not let go. He claimed that they were never even sexual, primarily because he knew he was not going to follow through with the relationship. But the woman turned out to have a history of stalking. She proceeded to call my client numerous times a day, and she would show up unannounced at his apartment and workplace. At times, neighbors had to call the police because the woman became violent. She once grabbed and scratched him and tore the shirt off his back. Even after the man obtained a restraining order, the women refused to stop pursuing him until the judge threatened to put her in jail. While the woman believed that she was only trying to salvage the short-lived relationship, she was in effect losing more and more control. Eventually the legal system officially ended the union.

It is well known that abused partners have a difficult time escaping. Some reasons for this are: (1) the victim may fear that leaving will only escalate abuse; (2) a lack of resources to support the victim's independence; (3) a lack of social and institutional support; and (4) because the cycle of abuse is deceiving. The cycle consists of three phases: *honeymoon phase*, *tension building phase*, and the *abuse phase*. Following the abuse phase, the abuser may express guilt and a willingness to change. This draws the victim back into the cycle, which only repeats itself (Women Against Abuse, 2021).

It is my belief that the internalized conflict plays a big role in holding people together even under the most abusive conditions. I have seen many individuals who appear to be grieving over the loss of an abusive relationship. But they are not necessarily grieving for the loss of the abusive partner as much as they are for the loss of their destructive dynamic. It is this dynamic that is employed to keep the conflict alive.

Codependency and Control: Caretaking and Enabling

Beattie (1986) defined codependency as a "person who has let another person's behavior affect him or her, and who is obsessed with controlling that person's behavior" (p. 1). According to Pikiewicz (2013), codependents are controlling because they lacked role models who demonstrated "appropriate" levels of responsibility in their youth. This in part, makes it difficult for them to set clear boundaries in adult relationships.

Caretaking and caregiving are considered concepts that exist on a continuum of codependency (Kupferman, 2010; Pikiewicz, 2013). Asa (2016) claimed that caretaking someone you perceive as needy can be a form of control. Whether the partner in need is developmentally limited, mentally, physically ill, or an addict, the caretaker or presumed healthier partner may take on the job of looking out for this person.

Caretakers are generally considered gentle, patient souls with high tolerance levels; those willing to give of themselves, often with little reward. But if the caretaking is chronic, almost obsessive, void of appropriate delegation and limit setting, the caretaker has lost perspective and is pursuing an objective that may be out of their conscious reach.

According to Kupferman (2010), caretakers are often stressed, they cross boundaries, do not practice self-care, are all knowing, and fail to delegate. Caregivers give happily, set clear boundaries and limits, delegate, and include the needy individual in the care process. The author claimed that a healthy dynamic involves a move from caretaking to caregiving.

Most chronic caretakers, especially those on the verge of burnout, are attempting to achieve a form of control. The type of control a person is looking for is particular to the person. Many are pursuing power. Others may be looking for approval, or to pay off a debt that is owed to their partner or to someone from their respective family of origin (Boszormenyi-Nagy & Spark, 1973). And some may be acting out the process of caring to avoid guilt or shame, which fits well with the paradoxical thesis of this book: that people simultaneously want and reject control.

Any caretaker who takes on irreparable projects, or who has unrealistic expectations even for a somewhat manageable project, is courting failure and ultimately, a lack of control. It will appear that the caretaker is in control. After all, the caretaker may control your medication, whether you get out of bed, and in some cases who you can have contact with. But most often the caretaker never fulfills their conscious objectives, and this is by unconscious design. Those who caretake attempt to control but rarely end up having any real sense of it. It is a fantasy that keeps their conflict alive.

Enabling has been defined as doing something for an individual that they can do themselves (Martin, 2020). Enabling is used commonly in the addictions field to represent an individual that consciously or unconsciously encourages or supports addictive behavior. But enabling can also refer to individuals in relationships that support any harmful or problematic behavior (Legg, 2019).

According to Martin (2020), enabling can be controlling because it is an attempt to control what someone else is doing or to control the outcome of a situation, even though it rarely works. The author concluded that although enablers see themselves as rescuers with good intentions, most help to thwart their partner's growth and ability to take responsibility. Martin also claimed that most enablers are simply trying to control their own anxiety.

Peter and Lisa were a married couple in their early 30s. Peter considered himself a liberal man and he never wanted to control Lisa in any way. He allowed her to socialize with her many girlfriends even though most were single, go to dance clubs without him, and to come home anytime she wanted. And she would sometimes return from these adventures in the early morning. For the most part, Peter refrained from asking any questions. But when he did, Lisa took little responsibility for her adolescent behavior and instead blamed him for acting like "her father." At a holiday block party, however, Lisa told Peter she was going for a walk with a male friend only to return hours later after the party had ended. Peter admitted that he felt somewhat humiliated, but only because a friend questioned his judgement on this matter. At another party, Lisa disappeared with the same male friend for over two hours. One day Peter came home from work and found this man and his wife in the living room. It was then that they admitted to

Peter they were in love and that Lisa was filing for divorce. Peter was in shock. While he was a genuinely nice man, and seemingly well-intentioned, he was a classic enabler in the context of his marriage.

Financial Control

Money makes the world go around: it feeds people, provides shelter, and can be used to educate children; it can be put to good use. But money can also be used as a class separator, and to get what one wants no matter how unethical or immoral. It can also be used to control one's partner. Some refer to this form of control as economic or financial abuse (Gordon, 2020; Smith, 2016; Steber, 2018). Smith (2016) wrote: "economic abuse occurs when one partner takes control of the other's financial life to gain power in the relationship."

Women are more prone than men to be the victims of financial control in their relationships. Sheey (2019) found that approximately 70% of millennial women felt as if they were financially controlled by their partners. One factor is that women are still paid less than men. According to PayScale (2021), when not controlling for compensatory factors, women make $0.82 for every dollar a man makes. When men and women with the same employment characteristics do similar jobs, women earn $0.98 for every dollar earned by an equivalent man. For more details on this issue see the section on sociocultural context in "Chapter 1. Control and Conflict."

A second factor is that many women still prefer the traditional role of staying home to raise the children. But regardless of what roles either partner chooses, neither should be dominated or controlled financially by the other unless one partner is clearly out-of-control financially. The following is an example of a couple in which one partner was controlling the other financially. Once again, notice how the control exerted by the husband over his wife eventually backfired. This case underscores the conflict about control.

Frank, a plumber in his late 50s, grew up poor courtesy of his parents' ineptness with money. "They made decent money, but they spent every penny they had. Then I had to support them until they passed. I promised myself I would not end up like them," he said. Given his experience, Frank said his main goal in life was to send his two daughters to college if they chose to go, and to have a healthy nest egg so that he and his wife, Joy, could enjoy an early retirement without burdening his children.

Frank was obsessed with money, and he brought the subject up in every session. He talked about how much he had, how much he was putting away, and what he would have by the time he reached 65-years old. Joy, a few years younger, claimed that Frank would micromanage her spending. Surprisingly, Frank admitted that Joy was not out-of-control, and in fact she was relatively frugal. But he thought she could do even better on a strict budget. When Joy went over her budget, she claimed that most of what she bought was for the kids. Frank disagreed and would berate her. It got to the point that Joy said she was afraid to spend a penny—even money that she earned from her part-time job.

According to Joy, if there were no financial surprises and Frank was on track with his retirement goal, he was tolerable. She did, however, say that if a major expense suddenly appeared, like needing a new water heater or refrigerator, Frank would sulk for weeks at a time. Frank agreed and said that every time he feels as if he is in control of the family's finances an unexpected expense appears. He said he seems to take three steps forward and four steps backwards.

Frank was not a mean man, but he was very controlling, especially in the context of money. After about four months of treatment, he was able to relax a bit knowing that unlike his parents, he was a saver who was too cautious to end up like them. But then something unexpected happened: Frank's financial advisor—an old friend from high school—called and told him that Joy lost a lot of money in the market. Apparently, Joy was trading behind his back. She wanted to make a quick buck to help with impending college expenses. Shocked, Frank could not believe what was happening. He said he felt betrayed and that he was not sure if he could ever trust Joy again. While Joy was guilty of deception, the money she was trying to earn was for a good cause. Her biggest problem, however, was her fear of Frank's rigid obsessiveness with money and her inability to openly express herself.

It took the better part of a year of treatment, but Frank came to see how his control was unproductive and had, in fact, backfired on him. He gained insight as to how struggles about money were ironically causing him to risk reaching his financial goals. To his credit, he decided to work with his wife rather than to financially dominate her. Joy struggled, but because she wanted to avoid a divorce, she worked hard to become more assertive. She admitted that she had a history of feeling guilty about saying "no" to anyone and had always felt sorry for her parents who mismanaged their money.

The following is an example of a couple in which the wife was a big spender and unlike Frank, the husband was not controlling by nature. In fact, he was too lax, until he had to intervene and take control. Bradley and Jill were a couple in their 40s. Bradley was a pleasant man who presented as naturally easy-going. But he was very frustrated that he could not convince his wife to curb her spending. Jill admitted that she spends a lot of money, but she was more concerned about being controlled than she was in negotiating a comprise with Bradley on her spending.

After several years, Bradley finally reached his breaking point. His business was slowing, and he worried that he would not have enough money to send his three children to college. His first move was to cut up all the couple's credit cards. He then pulled a large sum of money out of their checking account and left just enough to pay the monthly bills. He followed this by investing the bulk of the couple's savings in his name so that Jill could not spend it. Bradley claimed that he did not want to do these things, but Jill left him no choice. He even offered to lighten the restrictions if Jill promised to go to gambler's anonymous or to see a psychiatrist. But Jill was in no mood to negotiate. She was irate. She simply saw Bradley as a "sexist, control freak." Within four months Jill began having an affair and by the end of the year she left Bradley for another man. She filed for divorce soon thereafter. Staying on for a few individual sessions after his work with Jill, Bradley expressed remorse and wondered whether he should have tried to control Jill. He said that he never saw himself as controlling and hated being so. But he soon concluded that he would have had to set limits at some point, and it was better to do so sooner than later.

Sexual Control

Using sex to try and control a partner's behavior is not uncommon, and not necessarily a bad thing. Flirting for example, can be manipulative and controlling but is essential for successful mating (Nicholson, 2020), building intimacy, conveying an investment in the relationship, and maintaining romance (Horan, 2012). Frisby and Booth-Butterfield (2012) found that it helps to create a "private world" for a couple. Flirtatious behavior can be problematic, however, when it is used as a weapon to create animosity or jealousy in a partner.

Janie was a woman in her 20s. As an erotic dancer, Janie had plenty of opportunity to meet a variety of men. Her boyfriend of four years, Tom, wanted Janie to leave her job and find something he felt was more conservative and less threatening to him. But he also had another reason: It seemed that every time Janie did not like something Tom said or did, she would take on more hours at her club. One evening when she knew Tom was coming to give her a ride home, she decided to give another man a lap dance in front of Tom. Tom became enraged and the couple had a big fight at the club and were told to leave. It was clear that Janie crossed a relationship boundary and when boundaries are crossed to control someone, serious problems often arise.

Problems also may arise when one partner attempts to control the other by withholding sex. Unfortunately, this is too often a problem in relationships and one that is seen quite frequently by couples and sex therapists. Most of the time the withholding is a conscious, retaliatory act by an angry or frustrated partner. But the withholding may also be unconscious. The following case illustrates sexual withholding:

Bill and Elenore were a couple in their late 40s. Bill had not initiated or participated in sex with his wife in the year prior to treatment. While Elenore accused Bill of being gay, having an affair, or suffering from a mental disorder, none were true. It turned out that Bill was struggling financially and even though he begged his wife several times to curb her spending, she refused to do so. Bill withheld sex to get her to finally pay attention to him. Unfortunately, he waited too long, and his wife left him.

Some individuals use sex to control in a far more destructive and pathological manner. Jantz (2015) contended that not all relationships are on equal footing. One individual may exercise control over the other and use this advantage in areas that are not theirs to control. Jantz refers to these individuals as sexual manipulators. He wrote:

> For a sexual manipulator, pursuit can be lengthy. Each encounter that produces a small concession on the part of the person under their control fuels their desire

and escalates their behavior. They may begin pursuit with overly personal comments about attire or appearance. These seemingly innocuous comments may be followed by increasingly specific, sexual references. These may begin with sexual jokes or comments used to gauge the other person's reactions. As the manipulator's behavior gradually becomes more sexually overt, the sensibility of the target may be blunted.

(p. 1)

Finally, in some patriarchal countries, sexual manipulation and control in intimate relationships is sanctioned. For example, in Afghanistan, women must acquiesce to their male counterpart's sexual demands. Other countries criminalize rape but not the rape of a spouse. Jordan, Saudi Arabia, Sri Lanka, and Tanzania are a few examples. Some countries consider the wife's age when deciding whether to criminalize marital rape. In India the rape of a spouse is illegal only if the bride is under the age of 15 years. In Singapore, marital rape is not against the law if the bride is over 13 years of age (Shugerman, 2019).

The value of something lies in the demand for it, and there has always been a great importance given to sex both on micro and macro levels. But great need also can create the opportunity for corruption, and sex has proven to be a worthy context (Foucault, 1990).

Techniques Used to Avoid Being Controlled

The following behaviors are techniques of "resistance" that are often used in many different relational processes and contexts, especially in the one most germane to this book: control struggles in long-term relationships. That is, these techniques can easily be used by partners in a way that represents one side of their control conflict: to avoid being controlled. Unfortunately, however, they also end up satisfying the other side—the one that evokes more control from their partner. I believe that these techniques are distinct enough to merit their own individual categories.

Avoidance (Distancing)

Avoidance is often used to escape from being controlled by one's partner. This form of distancing, however, is commonly known to provoke the partner's need to pursue—as is depicted in the *pursuer-distancer* dynamic (Betchen, 2005; Fogarty, 1979). In fact, many of the clinical cases illustrated in "Chapter 6. Treatment Techniques for Couples with Control Struggles," resemble the complementary pursuer-distancer dynamic.

Avoidance or distancing may come in many forms. One male client worked long hours as a newspaper editor and never missed an opportunity to work overtime. While he claimed that his boss wanted him to put in the extra hours, in speaking with the wife of her husband's boss, she was told the complete opposite: the boss thought her husband should spend more time with his family. Another form of distancing used commonly by younger male partners is to fill their lives with activities that only they enjoy. For example, I have seen many young men who continue to play sports well into their 40s and 50s. One such man played soccer in high school and continued to do so after he was married. While not a problem in of itself, much to his wife's chagrin, the man joined one team after another and ended up playing all year round. She sarcastically told him that she would like her freedom to pursue a "real man."

While some partners might lean towards using work and hobbies to distance, others prefer using their friends or children. For example, one male client complained to me that his wife had many friends and seemed to prefer their company to his. He was a rather pleasant guy but was hurt and disappointed. His wife claimed that her behavior was harmless and that her husband should join she and her friends; but she was insincere. For the most part she and her friends shopped for hours and then lunched; she knew her husband would not be able to tolerate this activity for too long a time. Although he tried, she was right.

Using the children to distance—consciously or unconsciously—from a partner is all too common, and potentially destructive to a relationship. In my clinical experience couples create child-centered marriages to ignore marital problems, make less effort towards romance, create a barrier to intimacy, have a sense of control, and to avoid making the mistakes their parents made. But if childcare and time for the marriage are not balanced, the marriage will suffer. For example, a male client with two daughters built a full basketball court behind his house. He had played the game in his youth and looked forward to the day his children would play with him. Although somewhat disappointed that he and his wife were unable to conceive boys, to their father's delight his two daughters played the game. The client's oldest daughter, a talented high-school player, was as obsessed about the game as he was. Every day after school and for many hours on weekends father and daughter played together. The father also coached his daughter in the off-season in a summer league.

While the client's wife initially thought it was wonderful that she was married to such an involved father, she soon began to complain about their restricted lifestyle:

> Everything revolves around my girls and this game. And because I do not play, I feel as if I am left out. My husband seems to have little interest in me. I think he is trying to stay away from me and using our kids. I think he would be satisfied living with them.

As problems in the marriage escalated, the wife threatened to divorce her husband unless he attended couples therapy with her. During treatment, the husband finally got up the courage to tell his wife that she put too much pressure on him to act like a "grown up." Apparently, she always had chores for him to do. He further claimed that his wife's anxiety about keeping the house clean and organized ruled his life. In this sense, he admitted running away from her to avoid her rigid schedule of adult responsibilities. As the couple tried to negotiate a balance of work and play, the wife had to face her obsessive rigidity.

Dismissive Behavior

There are several ways to dismiss your partner and in turn, attempt to ward off being controlled. Everybody at one time or another has experienced someone literally waving off one of their comments with a hand gesture. It is as they are rejecting your idea or message without consideration. Most times their response is meant to avoid getting involved, but it is often taken as: "I am not interested in your perspective" or "That is the dumbest thing I have ever heard." Other times the partner may simply give short shrift or minimize your point. Examples of this are: "Just get over it" or "You're making too big a deal out of it."

"Eye rolling" is another common dismissive technique. Cameron, a man in his early 50s complained that unless his wife agreed with him, she would roll her eyes and walk away. Cameron claimed that he wanted his wife to stay and negotiate but that she would always shut down too soon, which often left him frustrated. Cameron's wife, Jackie, claimed that Cameron was a "control freak" and that the only reason he wanted to have a discussion was to beat her into submission and to have his way. To counteract his control, Jackie employed the eye rolling technique which she said she learned from her mother.

"Feigning deafness" is an effective technique for avoiding control. Acting as if you did not hear your partner can be a convenient alibi—one that can confuse your partner: "Does he hear me or is he having hearing problems?" A female client found that whenever her husband did not want to do the chores, he would turn down his hearing aid. She even went as far as to recommend he make an appointment with an audiologist to have his hearing aid tested.

Dismissive behavior can be accompanied by a grunt, sigh, or some other sound that emphasizes a lack of interest in being asked to engage. If you ask any person with experience what it feels like to have been dismissed, they will tell you that it made them feel as if they did not matter. This supports Bonior's (2016) contention that a dismissive response is an invalidating maneuver which: "creates an environment where it feels unwelcome and unsupported to express even the most understandable of human reactions" (p. 1).

To avoid control is not the only reason partners dismiss each other. They may do so out of anger or to antagonize (Higgens, 2016), or because of a deep fear of intimacy (Shorey, 2018). Regardless of the reason or the style employed, Becker-Phelps (2019) claimed that a dismissive response may only make the relationship dynamics worse.

Procrastination

Steel and Klingsieck (2015) defined procrastination as "a pervasive and pathological delay, where we put off despite expecting to be worse off" (p. 1). Ferrari (2010) found that procrastination is not about poor time management as some believe, but rather a self-sabotaging behavior rooted in a fear of failure, fear of success, and thrill-seeking. I have seen procrastination used in intimate relationships to avoid being controlled, even when the behavior seriously threatened the viability of the relationship—which it often does. Unlike the partner who feigns deafness, the procrastinator usually makes a verbal promise to submit to a partner's wishes, but rarely comes through in a timely fashion, if ever. Some procrastinators believe that they intend to carry out a partner's wishes but simply forget to do so. Others claim to have too little time. Much of this resistance is unconscious; others are consciously ambivalent and would rather control the situation themselves.

Ted, 58, owned and operated his own business. His wife Teresa held a full-time job in an insurance company as an underwriter. Teresa said that their home needed repairs which Ted could easily fix, but that he has put them off for years. She also claimed that Ted had plenty of time to take on some of these domestic tasks, but he usually spent every weekend watching television. Teresa said that she would gladly help but that Ted puts her off and keeps making promises he never keeps.

Ted admitted that he was a television addict, but he also offered that in the past, he has tried to keep up with his wife's demands but that the tasks kept coming. Ted said that he soon realized that his wife always needed to be engaged in a project and that by giving her control he would be working around the clock and never have a life. Ted was right about his wife, but not to the extent that he claimed. With the help of treatment, once the couple agreed on which tasks to tackle, their marital strife dissipated.

Passive-Aggressive Behavior

According to Parrot (2018), passive-aggressive behavior is always harmful, but especially so in marriage. Lancer (2017) claimed that passive-aggressive partners may act passive but are covertly expressing their negative feelings. They are basically obstructionist and their unconscious anger is projected onto each other. Clinicians (Meyer, 2020; Whitson, 2016) have found that in relationships, passive-aggressiveness may manifest in withdrawing behavior, procrastination, pretending a situation is all good when it is far from it, and doing things inefficiently or incompletely.

In my extensive work with couples, I have found that some partners become angry when they feel their mates try to control them. Fearing a blowup, they withhold their anger only to act out passive-aggressively. One of the most common passive-aggressive behaviors is to block the controller at every step. The following is an example of what this can look like in a marriage and how it can evolve into a control struggle.

Adam, 53, was a classic passive-aggressive partner. He grew up with parents who rarely asked anything of him and became quite resentful later in life when others did. In fact, he admitted in treatment that he took great pleasure in rebelling against people who he thought were ordering him around. Adam somehow managed to barely get himself through college with the help of a few generous professors, but once he married, he was in constant trouble.

Adam's wife, Marcy, was an organized, responsible woman with a somewhat dominant streak. She was the perfect foil for Adam's passive aggressiveness. Whatever Marcy asked Adam to take on, he either pleaded incompetence, said he would do it and forget, or say he would and do such a terrible job that she had too re-do it. For example, Adam resented picking the children up after school, but he would not voice this to Marcy. Instead, he would either pick them up much later than agreed or fail to get them at all. Once he left them waiting after school in the rain. Adam was also unreliable when it came to holding down a job and paying household bills. Whenever he felt that a company was charging too much, he would either pay half the bill . . . late, or not at all. His wife hated paying late fees, but Adam did not seem to mind.

One of Adam's favorite tricks that was especially infuriating to Marcy was his tendency to turn his cell phone off when it was not in use. He admitted that this prevented Marcy from being able to put pressure on him. Marcy said that felt as if she had another child to look after. Because Marcy no longer saw Adam as a responsible man, she lost all sexual interest in him. This in turn angered Adam, but he kept it bottled up inside which in turn, increased his passive-aggressive behavior. When Marcy finally left Adam, he had a great deal of difficulty understanding what happened. Adam was adept at blocking his wife or anyone else from controlling him.

Addictive Behavior

According to the National Center for Drug Abuse Statistics (NCDAS) (2021), 14.8 million people in the United States (aged 12 and over) struggled with an alcohol disorder, and 8.1 million with an illicit drug disorder. As many as 10 million people have a gambling addiction (North American Foundation for Gambling Addiction, 2016), and the number of people with a sex addiction is estimated at 12 million (Greenlaw, 2019).

Addicts are focused on whatever they are addicted to, whether it be alcohol, drugs, gambling, or sex. The addiction is number one in their lives and everything else including family, friends, and work come after. Many addicts are very conscious of this and use the addiction as an escape from the control of others who hold them responsible for their behaviors, especially their partners. Ask any partner how hard it is to control an addict and they will tell you stories of failure and frustration.

Addicts are secretive, and most lie (Hartney, 2019). As a result, their partners never know the whole truth about what they are up to—an effective way to avoid being controlled. A female client told me that after her ex-husband had finally moved out of the family home, she found an almost endless number of empty whiskey and wine bottles hidden in her basement. She said that she knew that her husband was an alcoholic, but she did not think the problem was as extreme as she discovered. Another female client only learned of the seriousness of her husband's gambling problem when she found that he had used their children's college savings to support his habit. When she confronted him, rather than show remorse he waved her off (dismissed her) by claiming that he had plenty of time to replenish their savings.

Addicts cause a lot of harm to themselves and those closest to them, but the fix is worth it to them. In fact, one of the characteristics that separate addicts from others is their willingness to take risks to feed their addiction. I have seen numerous sex addicts who did not even consider using condoms during the height of the AIDs crisis. Others have repeatedly cheated on their partners and spent an inordinate amount of money on porn usage. One man paid escorts to come to his home when his wife was away. When a neighbor questioned him, the man claimed that they were maids.

The stories about alcoholics and drug addicts are legendary. A gambling addiction, for example, can create incredible stress on the gambler and his or her family. A male client I saw attributed his early heart attack to being thousands of dollars in debt. He even had to pawn his wife's wedding ring several times over. When he gambled away the money that he had borrowed and could not pay it back, he feared his lenders would retaliate and harm his family. He believed this stress caused him to pass out at work. Later he found out he had suffered a heart attack. He was 42-years old with no family history of heart disease.

Most addicts become upset with those who try to interfere with their addiction. Ironically, however, many have a radar-like ability to mate with an enabler or someone who will tolerate and support their addiction. Perhaps most germane to conflict theory they, consciously or unconsciously, seek out rescuers or people that will move heaven and earth to try to help them beat their addiction, usually to no avail. One of the major reasons the failure rate is so high is because the addict is in conflict about being helped. They want to be in control of themselves and their addiction and choose a partner ostensibly to help them achieve this state. On the other hand, they want to maintain their addiction and the high it brings, no matter how chaotic and out-of-control life gets. Other addicts demonstrate this by marrying an addict. This way nobody interferes with the addiction process unless one partner decides to make a change.

References

Asa, R. (2016, August 11). *When caretaking gives you too much control.* YourCareEverywhere. www.yourcareeverywhere.com/caregiver-center/when-caretaking-gives-you-too-much-control.html

Beattie, M. (1986). *Codependent no more: How to stop controlling others and start caring for yourself.* Hazelden.

Becker-Phelps, L. (2019, January 16). *When your partner is dismissive.* WebMD. drbecker-phelps.com/home/when-your-partner-is-dismissive/

Betchen, S. (2005). *Intrusive partners-elusive mates: The pursuer distancer dynamic in couples.* Routledge.

Bonior, A. (2016, March 8). 5 behaviors no one in a relationship should accept. *Psychology Today*. www.psychologytoday.com/us/blog/friendship-20/201803/5-behaviors-no-one-in-relationship-should-accept

Boszormenyi-Nagy, I., & Spark, G. (1973). *Invisible loyalties*. Harper & Row.

Brogaard, B. (2015, March 27). 15 disturbing forms of verbal abuse in relationships: The abuser feels more powerful when he puts down his victim. *Psychology Today*. www.psychologytoday.com/us/blog/the-mysteries-love/201503/15-disturbing-forms-verbal-abuse-in-relationship

Center for Disease Control and Prevention (2021). *The National Intimate Partner and Sexual Violence Survey (NISVS)*. Retrieved July 28, 2021, from www.cdc.gov/violenceprevention/datasources/nisvs/index.html

Ferrari, J. (2010). *Still procrastinating*. Wiley.

Fogarty, T. (1979). The distancer and the pursuer. *The Family*, *7*, 11–16.

Foucault, M. (1990). *The history of sexuality, Vol. 1: An introduction* (R. Hurley, Trans.; 2nd ed.). Vintage (Originally work published 1976).

Frisby, B.N., & Booth-Butterfield, M. (2012). The "how" and "Why" of flirtatious communication between marital partners. *Communication Quarterly*, *60*, 465–480. https://doi.org/10.101080/01463373.2012.704568

Gordon, S. (2020, May 6). *How to identify financial abuse in a relationship*. Verywellmind. www.verywellmind.com/financial-abuse-4155224

Gottman, J., & Silver, N. (2015). *The seven principles for making marriage work* (rev. ed.). Harmony.

Greenlaw, E. (2019, January 15). *Understanding sex addiction*. Healthgrades. www.healthgrades.com/right-care/substance-abuse-and-addiction/understanding-sex-addiction

Hartney, E. (2019, June 29). *Why addicts lie even to loved ones*. Verywellmind. www.verywellmind.com/my-addicted-loved-one-lies-all-the-time-22118

Higgens, M. (2016, February 4). *6 signs you might be dismissive of your partner*. Bustle. www.bustle.com/articles/139688-6-ways-you-might-be-dismissing-your-partner-without-even-realizing-it.

Horan, S. (2012, August 16). Reasons people flirt. *Psychology Today*. www.psychologytoday.com/us/blog/adventures-in-dating/201208/reasons-people-flirt

Jantz, G. (2015, May 19). How to identify a sexual manipulator. *Psychology Today*. www.psycholgytoday.com/us/blog/hope-relationships/201505/how-identify-sexual-manipulator

Kupferman, E. (2010, February 10). *Codependency: Caretaking and caregiving*. Expressive Counseling. www.expressivecounseling.com/articles/codependency-caretaking

Lancer, D. (2017, June 20). Is your partner passive-aggressive? *Psychology Today*. www.psychologytoday.com/us/blog/toxic-relationships/201706/is-your-partner-passive-aggressive

Legg, T. (2019, June 27). *What is an enabler? 11 ways to recognize one*. National Alliance on Mental Illness. https://www.healthline.com/health/enabler

Martin, S. (2020). *How to stop enabling*. https://livewellwithsharonmartin.com/stop-enabling/

Meyer, C. (2020, December 21). *How to recognize signs of passive aggressive behavior in your spouse*. Brides. mydomaine.com/passive-aggressive-behaviors-in-marriage-1102423

National Center for Drug Abuse Statistics (2021). Retrieved from July 28, 2021, from www.drugabusestatistics.org

Nicholson, J. (2020, December 11). What is your flirting style? How do you flirt? *Psychology Today*. www.psychologytoday.com/us/blog/the-attraction-doctor/202012/what-is-your-flirting-style-how-do-you-flirt.

North American Foundation for Gambling Addiction (2016). Retrieved July 28, 2021, from https://nafgah.org/statistics-gambling-addiction-2016/

Parrot, L. (2018, March 14). *5 ways to cope with a passive-aggressive spouse*. SYMBIS Assessment. www.symbis.com/blog/5-ways-to-cope-with-a-passive-aggressive-spouse/

PayScale (2021). *The state of the gender pay gap 2021*. Retrieved July 28, 2021, from www. payscale.com/compensation-today/2021/02/payscale-releases-cbpr-2021

Pikiewicz, K. (2013, July 26). "Codependent" no more? *Psychology Today*. www.psychologytoday. com/us/blog/meaningful-you/201307/codependent-no-more

Sheey, K. (2019, October 10). Financial abuse: 70% of millennial women say partner used. money for control. *NYPost*. https://nypost.com/2019/10/08/nearly-70-of-millennial-women-financially-abused-by-partner/

Shorey, H. (2018, February 6). Dismissing attachment and the search for love. *Psychology Today*. www.psychologytoday.com/us/blog/the-freedom-change/201802/dismissing-attachment-and-the-search-love

Shugerman, E. (2019, March 26). *There are still 10 countries where it is legal to rape your spouse*. REVELIST. www.revelist.com/user/EmilyShugerman

Smith, A.K. (2016, August 10). *How money is used as a weapon in relationships: Financial literacy is a key to fighting economic abuse*. Kiplinger. www.kiplinger.com/article/spending/t065-c023-s002-how-money-is-used-as-a-weapon-in-relationships.html

Steber, C. (2018, May 21). If your partner does these 11 things, it may be financial abuse. *Bustle*. www. bustle.com/p/if-your-partner-does-these-11-things-it-may-be-financial-abuse-10139159

Steel, P., & Klingsieck, K. (2015). Procrastination. In J.D. Wright (Ed.), *International encyclopedia of the social & behavioral sciences* (2nd ed., Vol. 19, pp. 73–78). Elsevier.

Whitson, S. (2016, October 18). Understanding passive aggressive behavior. *Psychology Today*. www.psychologytoday.com/us/blog/passive-aggressive-diaries/201610/understanding-passive-aggressive-behavior?

Wise, A. (2020, February 20). 5 sneaky reasons you are crying all the time: Not all tears are the same. *HuffPost*. www.huffpost.com/entry/why-youre-crying_n_5a26e553e4b06d807b4fa42c

Women Against Abuse (2021). *Why it is so difficult to leave*. Women Against Abuse. www. womenagainstabuse.org/education-resources/learn-about-abuse/why-its-so-difficult-to-leave

Wong, B. (2019, Aril 5). If you tend to cry during arguments: Here is why (and how to manage it). *HuffPost*. www.huffpost.com/entry/how-to-stop-crying-arguments_l_5ca4fa07e4b0ed0d7810256

Zoppi, C. (2020, November 11). *Why might a person cry for no reason?* MedicalNewsToday. www.medicalnewstoday.com/articles/crying-for-no-reason

Section II

Clinical Assessment

5 Assessing Couples With Control Struggles

The Initial Contact

The assessment phase begins when the couples therapist first receives a telephone call or email from one of the partners. If a couple has a conflict around control, the initiating partner may attempt to gain control over the clinician and the therapy before the first session. One technique used prior to treatment is to demand certain action or information from the therapist that would support the initial contact's perspective. For example, before we ever met, a female client told me that her husband had a history of porn usage. She then began to pressure me to advise her whether to take his computer from him. But I immediately countered that it is my policy not to offer any interventions until I get to know a couple. Setting limits and establishing clear boundaries immediately is an important way to battle control and create an organized, productive, and structured therapeutic environment (Weeks & Fife, 2014; Weeks et al., 2005).

The initiator of treatment may also question the therapist about the treatment approach. This is understandable if the questions are general in nature: Do you assign home exercises? Will you give us a book to read? But some clients demand that the therapist explain the therapeutic approach in detail even though most do not have the proper background to assess it. It is best to give a brief overview of your model knowing full well that the client's objective might be to increase their sense of control and to reduce yours. For example, a male client told me that he was interested in Imago therapy (Hendrix & Hunt, 2019). I politely told him that I know of the Imago approach and while there are some similarities between my model and Imago, I did not feel qualified to use that model. I also offered to refer him to somebody who does. Rather than take my referral, however, the man continued to pressure me to read a book on the subject; he was trying to assert control. When I refused and questioned him as to why he did not initially find an Imago therapist he had no answer but stayed on and allowed me to complete my assessment.

While some therapists recommend that a couple question a prospective therapist's credentials (Benson, 2020), this could be used as another control tactic: What degrees do you have? Where did you go to school? How many years have you been practicing? One man, a lawyer, asked me who I studied under—as if he

DOI: 10.4324/9781003159100-7

would know of these people. It turned out the only therapist he had ever heard of was Freud. Others have questioned my choice of degrees and program of study.

Under these conditions a therapist must stay calm and maintain a neutral stance. Some therapists experience anger or insecurity. But the therapist must have confidence in his/her ability and training and not take the probing personally; it is usually only a defense against the anxiety that often comes with change. Couples usually take some care in hiring a therapist. A recommendation from a friend or someone who has had a good experience with the therapist buys some good will in the therapeutic process.

But even if an insurance company has made the referral, a couple can check the clinician's credentials on the Internet or via a professional organization. All this is to say, a couple usually knows the therapist's credentials prior to assessment and so the questioning of credentials is a weak defense. If, under these conditions I cannot appease a client, I will again offer a referral. My experience is that this counter-maneuver often scares the client enough to back down; sometimes it provokes the non-initiating client into action to save the treatment.

The initiating partner may also follow up the first contact by sending a lengthy email or letter detailing the couple's entire history. Some people have sent me timelines from the first time they met to the present. While this may only happen once during treatment, some partners try to continue this form of communique to connect more closely to the therapist, unbalance the couple and skew the system in their favor, or to stretch out the therapy. If this occurs, the couple's therapist must set appropriate limits with the initiator as soon as possible or the behavior will probably continue. Gray (2006) contended that the therapist should always explain the reasoning behind setting limits in treatment. I usually tell the initiator that it is unfair to their partner to imbalance the treatment and it may even backfire and give the non-initiating partner a legitimate reason to prematurely end treatment.

The Chief Complaint

Nearly every therapist asks the couple why they are seeking treatment. While this information is often ascertained at the initial point of contact, via telephone or email, some therapists wait until the first session to see if the partners agree. The specific problem that the couple usually cites is commonly known as the presenting problem or chief complaint. I tend to take the couple's chief complaint at face value, but I generally think of it as the symptom of an underlying conflict rather than the cause of the couple's difficulty.

Some chief complaints are indicative of a conflict around control. For example, if a couple seeks treatment because of chronic fighting, it may be because the partners are locked into a struggle for control with no solution in sight. Bill and Kathy are an example of a couple that seem to fight over everything, big and small. In their late 40s, Bill and Kathy seemed to differ as a way of life. For example, the couple disagreed on big ticket items such as how much to spend on college tuition for their daughter. But by contrast, one of their most significant arguments was over the shades in the living room. Kathy enjoyed the sun and light and Bill preferred the dark. Kathy and Bill would take turns raising and lowering the shades and fighting each time a change was made.

Other couples may be gridlocked over one specific issue. These couples, for example, might present with a significant, contextual problem such as where to send the kids to school, or where to live. Janelle and Thomas were in their early 30s. Janelle was born and raised in the Northeast and wanted to remain there and start a family. Her parents and grandparents were still there as well as her siblings and she envisioned having plenty of support in raising children. She also liked city life and the four seasons.

Thomas longed to move to Arizona. He felt the Northeast part of the United States was flooded with people and that his career would flourish in the West. The couple fought incessantly over this but maintained their relationship. Approximately six weeks before their marriage they reached a compromise. They escaped gridlock by agreeing to move to Arizona. But the stipulations were that Janelle be allowed to fly home whenever she chose, and if she could not acclimate after two years the couple would return to the Northeast. They put off marriage until they were sure that their compromise was working.

The First Session

One partner, usually the initiator, may show up to the first session well before the significant other. This may be a tactic to get the therapist's sole attention, join with the therapist, and to slip in a few complaints about the partner. But the absent or late partner may not be innocent. He/she could be passively colluding—consciously or unconsciously—to set the therapist up to lose systemic balance. Most couples therapists make the smart choice and refuse treatment until both partners are present. This stance counters the client's attempt to take control and helps to maintain the integrity and balance of the couple system.

When one partner is late to the session, some couples therapists make the mistake of starting with the partner who is on time. These clinicians have told me that they feel guilty not giving the couple their full session time. Although there is something to learn from all client behavior, the therapist must hold "the couple" accountable for the lateness and grant no extra time. They chose each other and blaming the late partner will only result in an unbalancing of the treatment and may lead to premature termination. At times like these, it is especially important for the couple's therapist to remember that if one partner has a conflict around control, the other one does as well, and this makes collusion inevitable.

Some clients make a habit of being late and it may be a passive form of control that fits nicely with the couple's relational dynamic. I usually ask if the late partner is late in other contexts, and how the partner who is usually on time feels about the lateness. The answer to this question may give the therapist a view of what the couple's relational dynamic looks like on an everyday basis.

Nevertheless, setting appropriate time limits will: (1) prevent the clinician from feeling taken advantage of; (2) offer the clinician a sense of control; (3) force the partner who is late to give in to the therapeutic process; and (4) stop the colluding partner from contributing to the other partner's attempt to control the treatment.

It is not unusual for a couple to spend the entire first session arguing about being in treatment. To counter this, I usually check the non-initiator's commitment to the relationship. If the commitment is not there, I suspect there may be a potential sabotaging pattern in the couple's relationship. In tune with Doherty and Harris's (2017), I perceive this "mixed-agenda" couple (p. 3) consisting of one partner "leaning in" and the other "leaning out" of the treatment and the relationship (p. 136).

I highlight the mixed-agenda and frame it as a problem that must be dealt with before we can all move forward. But I also normalize it as part of the treatment process. Often the main blockage comes from the pressure the leaning-in partner is exerting on the process; they might want a guarantee that all will be well. I empathize with the leaning-in partner's anxiety and lack of control, but I also balance the treatment by pointing out that no one can truly predict the outcome of couples therapy. Demanding that the leaning-out partner guarantee therapeutic success would be somewhat unrealistic, and destructively premature.

I request that the leaning-out partner give the treatment a chance. But I also realize that this partner may merit the help of individual therapy to do so. This recommendation should be made judiciously because separating the couple might vastly increase the leaning-in partner's anxiety and has not been proven to be effective for couples problems (Gurman & Burton, 2014). The noncommitted or leaning-out partner may have to decide which is more important: holding out and refusing couple's work or risk losing the relationship. Ironically, the committed or leaning-in partner's position may be more difficult because this partner might have to decide whether to continue the relationship with a reluctant counterpart. Regardless, the couple's conflict around control will likely show itself early in the therapy.

I have been asked by many students whether they should pursue the reluctant partner on behalf of the initiator. The answer to this is almost always no: unless in a crisis, such as a potential suicide, never pursue a distancer (Betchen, 2005). This would put you in the same position as the pursuer and in turn, unbalance the couple system. It also enables the initiator and takes pressure off the couple to change their dynamic.

It may be the case that one partner does not want to attend treatment but does so under the threat of divorce. While this partner may simply fear losing control in the treatment process, he/she might resent being bullied into attending sessions. Sometimes there is a control struggle over the choice of therapist. A female client chose me for couples therapy, but over her husband's protest. The husband was so mad that his wife took control that he sabotaged the treatment by continuously complaining about the fee. The reality was that the husband did not care who the therapist was. What bothered him most was that his wife dictated the choice. If I spot this in the assessment phase, I address it immediately because I know that treatment will not go far under these conditions.

It is the couple's responsibility to agree on which therapist to hire before stepping into an office. While it is possible that the fit between couple and therapist might be a bad one, I specifically address this before we even meet. For example, a couple from another state wanted to commute over two hours by car to see me and I just did not think they would be able to follow through; I also saw it as a burden on the couple. I therefore recommended someone I knew in their vicinity.

If a couple proves committed enough for treatment, the first step many therapists take is to do an extensive assessment. Some clinicians prefer a more flexible approach and ask only a few key questions related to the couple's chief complaint. These therapists claim to take a session or two to "join" with the couple rather than risk premature termination. Some of these therapists fear going in too deep too soon or asking to many personal questions, especially of a sexual nature, before building a secure rapport with the couple (Weeks & Fife, 2014). This stance is especially taken by therapists who deal with particularly sensitive issues such as sexual abuse. However, in some instances a couple's sensitivity can be used as a defense against having to talk about uncomfortable material. It is normal for a previously abused partner to refuse to discuss their abuse, but if this resistance persists, and is supported by the seemingly empathic partner, a collusion might be evident. This may be especially true if the couple presents with a sexual disorder but refuses to discuss their sexual history.

In most cases, I prefer to get as much information as quickly as possible. The faster I can develop a working hypothesis about the couple's problem, the more quickly I can intervene. Once the treatment has started, it is usually harder for the therapist to go back and ask historical questions. This is because couples are anxious when they come for treatment and most prefer to look forward not backwards.

Another reason to do a formal assessment as soon as possible is because once a couple settles into their process or interactional dynamic, they are harder to stop long enough to complete an extensive assessment. Couples usually replay their dynamic and if allowed to do so for too long, they may feel as hopeless about the treatment as they already feel about their problem. When the couple's therapist takes charge of the therapeutic process, he/she is setting the structure of the treatment. The therapist is letting the couple know who is in charge. It also interrupts their natural chaotic flow.

While certain factors discovered in the initial contact can help the couple's therapist determine whether a control struggle is at play, more data is needed. I usually begin the formal assessment phase in the first session by drawing two connecting genograms (Bowen, 1978; DeMaria et al., 2017) in my notes. I then choose a partner to question, and I do not move onto the next partner until I have completed my questioning of the first partner. I choose to begin with the least resistant client; this allows the somewhat reluctant partner time to acclimate to the therapeutic process.

Some colleagues and students have questioned whether my style unbalances the treatment. That is a legitimate question. But I make sure that I give equal time to each partner even if the questioning flows over into the second session. I find value in requiring each partner to listen to the other's story and to add anything of significance that may have been missed. I believe that this assessment style may help to increase insight and build mutual empathy. I am also better able to form an alliance with each partner (Friedlander et al., 2018). This format sets the structure for treatment by conveying the message that each partner will be held responsible for their individual contributions to the relational problems.

My style may also expose a couple's control struggle if one partner refuses to answer basic questions about their family of origin. I often hear, "I do not want to blame my parents for this." Another tactic is to question the validity of my question or statements. When I questioned a male client's need for control in his marriage he responded: "That is just plain stupid." As treatment progressed, he placed everything I said in the same basic category—dumb and dumber.

Often, one partner tries to control or dominate the treatment, and this usually shows in the assessment phase. Some do so by talking so much that no one else, including the therapist, can get a word in. Before intervening, it would prove valuable for the therapist to see how the more passive partner handles this situation. Does this partner attempt to intervene and be heard or sit by passively and enable their counterpart to disrupt the therapeutic process? If the passive partner chooses to enable, the therapist should firmly but gently interrupt the controlling partner and put pressure on the passive partner by asking if he/she has any thoughts or feelings or opinions about what is being said. If this fails to provoke the passive partner, the therapist can add that the passive partner must not think they have anything important to add. If all else fails, the therapist should interrupt the controlling partner and let both partners know that they will not progress if this continues. I have offered the question: Why don't you let me help you?

One male client would not allow me or his wife to speak and challenging him only backed him off temporarily. His wife pleaded with him to let her voice her opinion but to no avail. When I told the husband that I could not help unless he let his wife speak, he gave me a commonly used reason for his behavior: "I am just trying to get you up to speed on our situation. I don't want to forget anything, and I think what I have to tell you is important." My response is usually: "I appreciate that, but I think I have a good picture of what is going on. Any more information will only shorten the time we have together. If I have any questions, I will be sure to ask you." I do not offer any deep interpretations or challenge the control struggle during the assessment phase. I prefer to stay focused on the gathering of data because the more information I get, the easier it will be to challenge the couple's defenses.

Questions for the Genogram

Many of the questions I ask during the assessment or intake phase have been presented in my previous work (Betchen & Davidson, 2018). But if the initial contact and couple's chief complaint suggests that a couple is experiencing an underlying conflict about control, I may add questions to determine its validity.

Because my approach is integrative, many of my questions are oriented towards a couple's sexual as well as nonsexual life. I almost always get a general picture of the couple's sexual relationship even if they present with a nonsexual symptom such as poor communication or chronic fighting. But if they present with a sexual symptom my sexual assessment is more comprehensive and detailed. Some of the questions I ask which might alert me that a nonsexual or sexual control struggle is at play are as follows:

When did you first start having this problem?
The longer a couple have had a problem, the more likely they have been in a control struggle.

Did you ever seek treatment for your problem before?
The more a couple has procrastinated in treating their problem, the more likely they have been in a control struggle.

Did you ever experience this problem in a previous relationship?
This might reveal a pattern of control struggles that precedes the current relationship.

Can you give me a detailed picture of your last sexual experience?
Kaplan (1995) would ask clients to give her a step-by-step or "video" picture of their most recent sexual experience (p. 96). I have found this concept useful in determining sexual gridlock. For example, you may find that while one partner is seducing, the other is looking at a cell phone. Another partner might be physically too rough or doing something the other partner clearly does not like. Asking this question might also be a great way to determine if one partner is sabotaging any prescriptive exercises the therapist has assigned.

Do you take any medications?
Medications may be used to cause or maintain a control struggle. For example, a partner with erectile disorder (ED) might refuse to fill his prescription for a medication and in turn, continue to fail to satisfy his partner. He might also sabotage when and how he takes it so that it will not be effective. For example, I have treated several men who have chosen to take ED drugs and wait only 20 minutes before attempting intercourse rather than the prescribed hour. This almost always ends in erectile failure.

Do you have any medical conditions?
Some medical conditions are inevitable, but if a partner refuses to treat it properly such as diabetes, it may provoke anger and frustration in their counterpart and in turn, a control struggle. This may also occur with the use and abuse of illegal drugs or alcohol.

Did you ever experience abuse of any kind?
According to Sewdayal (2021), traumatic past experiences can lead to a need for control in adulthood. If a person was abused emotionally, physically, or sexually, this individual may have developed a need to control in real time. I happened

to be treating a young woman in a clinic who had been sexually abused as a child when suddenly the lights went out. The young woman panicked so badly that she began to hyperventilate. I could not calm her until the lights went on. Apparently, her uncle held a dark sweater over her head as he molested her in her darkened bedroom. She admitted that she feels very out-of-control without light. She sleeps with her bedroom lights on.

When did you lose your virginity?
If too young, this might be a sign of impulsiveness or a lack of control.

Do you have siblings?
Having had controlling older siblings could result in a need for more control as an adult. Conversely, having been parentified by younger siblings, or having siblings with disabilities or chronic ailments may yield the same results (Boszormenyi-Nagy & Spark, 1973). Toman (1976) found that oldest siblings were more prone to having been given more control and responsibility when growing up.

Do any of your siblings have the same problem you do?
A need for control may run in siblings, given they came from the same household.

How would you describe your parent's relationship?
Witnessing control struggles when growing up may manifest into a familiar way of life.

Did one parent seem to always be upset with the other?
This can be an indirect way to find out if there were chronic control struggles in the family.

Did you favor a parent?
Empathizing with a particular parent may reveal your style of control. Specifically, you may have role modeled a perceived good parent's controlling style or rebelled against the perceived bad parent's style.

Did your parents approve of your relationship?
This is a common context for control struggles—especially, for example, if your relationship is interracial or interreligious. In many of my cases the point of contention between couple and parents is because of racial, religious, or socio-economic disparities.

Do you and your partner share similar interests, politics, values, religious and cultural backgrounds?
Lee (2013) and others (Lee & Park, 2013; Moodley et al., 2015; Sue & Sue, 2015) contend that understanding the role of culture, ethnicity, race, religion, sexual orientation, and experience with discrimination, is necessary to join with and accurately assess couples. Couples can easily experience struggles over any number of these issues. Many couples have currently found themselves gridlocked because of political differences, especially given our divided political atmosphere (Betchen, 2020).

What role did you play while growing up in your family?
If you had a controlling role in your family of origin you may be replicating it in your current relationship. Again, those children that were given the role of mediators or were parentified have more responsibility and therefore may transmit this control into adulthood (Boszormenyi-Nagy & Spark, 1973).

Did your parents talk about sex when you were a child?
If your parents were close-minded, you might have a greater tendency to control yourself and others. Often there is a punishment waiting for the family member who fails to comply with the rules of a closed system. In some cases, the open family member is heavily criticized or even alienated by family members because of their curiosity. This is often considered outside the lines of a closed family.

Do you masturbate?
Masturbation represents the ability to experience pleasure and sexual freedom independent of a partner. But if parents were critical of this activity, the act can later serve as a convenient context for a control struggle in adulthood by your substituting the activity for partner relations (Betchen, 1991).

Do you fantasize?
Allowing yourself to fantasize may be a sign of openness and personal freedom. It has also been shown to increase sexual desire (Birnbaum et al., 2018). If you cannot fantasize, it may indicate that you are controlling or repressing yourself.

Do you watch porn?
Another possible sign of personal freedom, porn usage, can be a positive, healthy, harm-free part of a couple's sex life. But some people partake in this activity enough to fuel relational dysfunction (Gonsalves, 2020) or a sexual control struggle. For example, some men may prefer porn to having sex with their wives (Betchen, 1991).

Do you have any paraphilias or fetishes?
Paraphilias (Brown, 2021) and fetishes (Angers, 2020) can negatively impact a relationship. These acts are often insatiable and persistent, and thus ripe for sexual gridlock. Some partners may be able to function without the use of their fetish and others may not. It is quite common for the partner of a fetishist to feel used or objectified, thus creating a sexual control struggle.

What type or form of sexual activity excites you the most?
Partners should express their sexual preferences or risk having an unfulfilling sex life. Poor communication can, in of itself, lead to sexual control struggles.

Are you physically attracted to your partner?
An underrated concept in our society is physical attraction. Many people are not physically attracted to their partners and yet try and maintain their relationships. Sometimes emotional and financial dependency are reasons for this, but the result is often sexual and emotional gridlock (Betchen, 2013b, 2015, 2019).

Are you sexually satisfied with your partner?
Many partners are unsatisfied with their partner's sexual prowess but are too afraid to address this issue. Holding these feelings back, however, may result in a control struggle either in a sexual or nonsexual context.

Did you ever consider having sex with someone of the same sexual orientation?
If you are not true to your identity or orientation, it will be easier to end up in a control struggle.

How often would you like to have sex?
It is not uncommon for a couple to disagree on this issue and as a result, become locked into a sexual control struggle (Watson, 2018). Some partners want sex every day and others once a month. The therapist need only focus on helping the couple break their gridlock and reach a compromise. Inflicting a value judgement is not necessary and will only unbalance the couple.

Do you have a sexually exclusive relationship?
Control struggles can develop if one partner wants an exclusive relationship and the other is in favor of polyamory or an alternate relationship form. Again, it is not the therapist's role to pass value judgements. It is, however, important that the therapist inform the couples of the potential consequences of their choices (Betchen, 2013a).

How long did you and your partner date before you formed an exclusive relationship?
An early indication of a budding control struggle is when partners never agreed when to become exclusive. The same can be said for having children.

To your knowledge, has there been any outside relationships or affairs?
To most, affairs are traumatic (Glass, 2021) and consequentially, a convenient context for control struggles. For example, the process that goes into deciding how and when to stop an affair is the perfect breeding ground for a control struggle.

Content Versus Process

Sometimes a couple present a symptom that is not necessarily indicative of a control struggle, but it may serve as the context or content for one. For example, if a couple present with Genito-Pelvic/Pain Penetration Disorder (GPPPD)—in which the female partner cannot allow for intercourse because of fear of vaginal penetration, vaginal pain during intercourse, and the tightening of vaginal muscles—I have found that the disorder may also be caused by an unconscious form of control. This may be especially true if the female is upset with her partner for any reason.

Exposing the underlying control struggle and its connection to a formidable symptom is usually not easy. To do so, the therapist must first be able to distinguish between *content* and *process* in the therapeutic setting. Content—used interchangeably with context—is the topic or subject matter that the couple disagree over. Content represents a couple's symptoms. In the previous example, the GPPPD would be the content; how the couple process this problem, or the underlying control struggle would be the process. Betchen and Davidson (2018) refer to content as the baggage that the process or vehicle carries.

To distinguish content and process the couple's therapist will have to carefully observe the couple from the beginning of treatment. Paying particular attention to how each partner interacts when dealing with their presented symptom as well as with issues across different contexts is important. This will be difficult because most couples want the clinician to focus on the chief complaint. In today's world where information is at everyone's fingertips, couples more than ever diagnose their problems and have an idea how to treat the problem. This can be both a good and a bad thing.

It is nice that people can more easily admit they have a problem and seek out professionals specifically qualified to treat it. But on more than one occasion, as previously mentioned, I have experienced clients who, having read about a disorder on the Internet, insist that I cure it in the exact amount of time referred to in the article or blog the client had consulted. Janet, for example, was right in diagnosing herself as having GPPPD, but she also told me that according to a blog she had read I should be able to alleviate the problem within 12 sessions.

The therapist and couple can take some comfort in knowing that the process rarely changes; but the content may vary. In the assessment phase, it is easy to understand why couples often feel overwhelmed—as if they have a host of problems with little hope of improvement. Being told that they have one problem (process) that can impact different contexts is often relieving to them. Nevertheless, the therapist should be aware when the chief complaint is alleviated, the process problem can show itself in a different context. Some therapists refer to this Freudian concept as "symptom substitution" (American Psychological Association, 2020). If a couple is warned that this could occur, they might not panic.

Couples may look as if they are simply struggling with an immediate behavioral issue, but an underlying conflict may be at play. For example, two partners can present their points of view calmly and rationally, serving to fool a therapist into thinking the case could be resolved with a behavioral intervention. However, this would have to be determined with caution. For example, Kent and his wife Tracy were a couple in their late 30s. Tracy wanted a third child, but Kent did not. Each partner presented their reasons in a polite manner making equally logical points. Tracy came from a small family which was spread all over the country. She did not want their daughter to grow up with only one sibling.

Kent acknowledged the value of Tracy's point but countered with his worry about finances and the couple's ability to care equally for more than two children given their demanding jobs. Apparently, their daughter also suffered from developmental disabilities, which both partners used to make their cases. Although this disagreement rarely escalated or seemed to threaten the couple's marriage, it had been going on for two years.

While some couples therapists may look to help this couple reach a compromise, with careful questioning I determined that the couple had never fully explored this issue before marriage. When one partner changes his/her mind about something this significant after marriage, a destructive control struggle often ensues. In this case, neither Kent nor Tracy clearly communicated how many children they each wanted prior to the marriage. It was only after they were married that each took an opposing stance on the matter. This highlights the point that a couple's control struggle may consciously or unconsciously begin early in the relationship only to cause problems at some later date.

A last example comes to mind. Within two months of the start of his exclusive relationship with Marsha, her husband Ari reported that Marsha became depressed and uninterested in having sex with him. Although Ari was disappointed, he took Marsha at face value and waited for her to get treatment for her depression. Following treatment, however, Marsha's sex drive failed to return. What Ari ignored is that Marsha never had much of a libido. Marsha was subconsciously aware that she was never that interested in having sex but had trouble admitting it to herself and to Ari. For his part, Ari, did not read between the lines. As soon as Marsha's depression lifted Ari saw—for the first time—that Marsha had a serious sexual problem that predated her depression. With her major excuse dissipated, a severe control struggle ensued which eventually led to the end of the relationship. Apparently, the struggle for control over sex had always been there. But the seriousness of it only showed itself after all other variables were controlled. The following examples are general illustrations of my assessment method with two couples in control struggles: one with nonsexual symptoms and the other with sexual symptoms.

Assessing Hank and Diane: A Nonsexual Control Struggle (See Figure 5.1)

Initial Contact and Chief Complaint

Diane first contacted me by telephone to tell me that she would like couples therapy for her and her husband of 18 years, Hank. Both partners were in their mid-40s. Diane reported that the couple needed help communicating because they were fighting constantly: her version of the couple's chief complaint. When asked what they usually fought about, Diane replied that their fights varied but were mostly over money. When asked how long they have been fighting, Diane answered that they always had disagreements but became more frequent and intense soon after they married and began earning more money. When asked which partner decided they needed help Diane said that she has been trying to get Hank into couples therapy for many years. She claimed the only reason Hank is now willing to attend is because she is threatening divorce.

Diane was brave enough to admit that she tried many times to get Hank to take her seriously, even having a brief fling years ago. But she said Hank is a

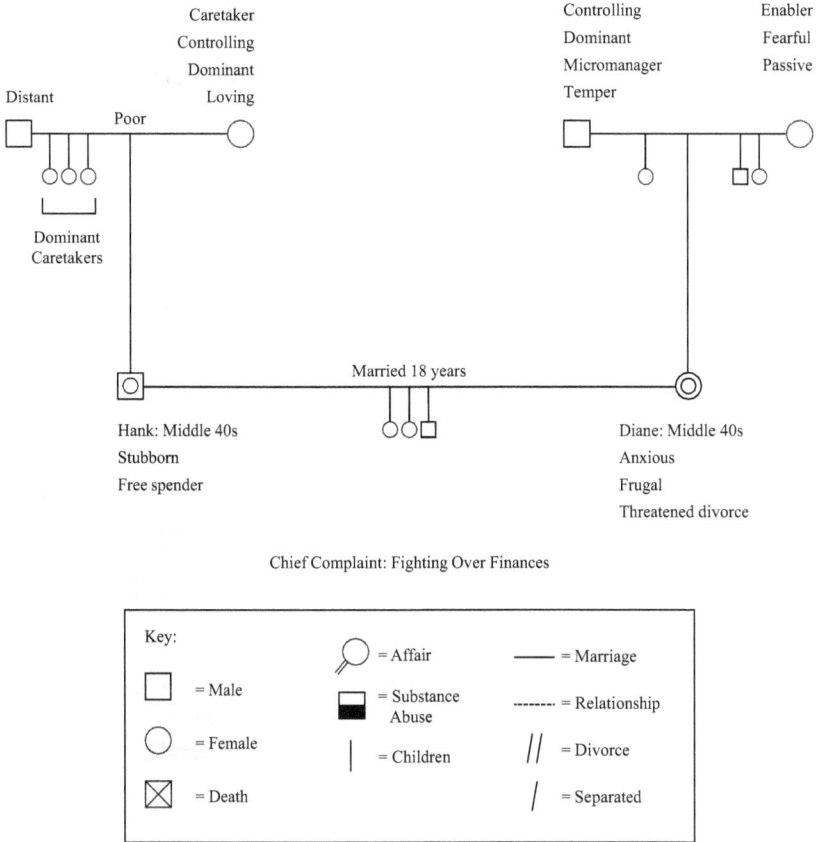

Figure 5.1   Hank and Diane.

stubborn man, and has become more challenging, even though he claims not to want a divorce.

First Session

In the first session, Hank confirmed that the couple fights frequently over money. But this is about the only thing he and Diane seemed to agree on. The information gleaned from the initial contact revealed that there was evidence that Hank and Diane were locked in a control struggle: frequent and longstanding disagreements in a variety of contexts which predated the couple's marriage; Diane's insistence on and Hank's resistance to treatment; and Hank's stubbornness coupled with Diane's anxiety. But to confirm this, I felt that more evidence was needed. I asked the couple to give me an example of one of their disagreements and to be as detailed as possible.

In my many years of supervising trainees, I have found that some therapists do not follow up a question with a request for an example of what the couple is talking about. I find this to be important for several reasons: (1) to give the therapist a clear picture of what is happening with the couple outside of the office setting; (2) to validate or invalidate what the couple is claiming; and (3) to better understand the way a couple is interpreting their relationship dynamics.

Diane told me of an incident in which the couple had a disagreement about finances. She said that Hank insisted that he wanted an inground swimming pool. He had always wanted a pool, but Diane felt their money would be better spent on fixing their home. The couple fought about this for nearly a year until one day Hank took control and purchased a pool. Diane complained that Hank acted as if he did not care what she thought. She was particularly enraged with Hank because she was the breadwinner in the family. Hank countered that he knew his wife's position, but he disagreed with her. He said the pool was for both to enjoy and that he was not going to let his wife control his spending. He felt that she was overanxious about many things and he did not want to live his life held hostage by her anxiety. Diane claimed that she takes a serotonin reuptake inhibitor (SSRI) to cope with Hank.

I did not take an extensive sexual history in this case because the couple did not suffer from any sexual disorders, and in fact, Diane reported their sex life has been more than adequate. While she was furious with Hank at times, she did not want to be one of those women who withheld sex. Diane claimed that she and Hank are still physically attracted to one another, but that she would leave him if things did not change. The following exchange will give you a feel for the level of hostility and gridlock in this marriage:

Diane: Hank doesn't care about my feelings. He knows that his spending habits make me anxious, but he does what he wants. Sometimes I have trouble sleeping because I never know what he'll want to buy next. And his tastes are expensive—they set us back. I want to retire comfortably and leave enough money for our two children to inherit. Hank doesn't seem to care about them either.

Hank: You're anxious about everything. What is the point of working so hard if we cannot enjoy life? Besides, we don't owe it to our kids to support them. We earned this money; let them earn their own.

Diane: I agree that we should enjoy life. But my idea of fun is not raiding our retirement and paying extra fees. I literally have an anxiety attack every time I hear from our accountant because I never know what new surprise awaits me. I just can't talk to you about this. You're impossible.

Therapist: Diane, have you two ever tried negotiating?

Diane: Hank doesn't negotiate.

Hank: I don't want to negotiate because what she really wants is to control everything.

Hank's accountant was on Diane's side on this one. To buy this pool Hank had to take money out of his retirement plan. He then had to pay a penalty and taxes for the withdraw. Hank also had a checkered financial history including a bankruptcy before he met Diane. In this sense, Hank's conflict around control was becoming more evident. While he was hell bent on not allowing Diane or anyone else to tell him what to do, many of his decisions were costly, and at times caused him serious difficulty. One incident that comes to mind was an altercation with a demanding boss. Hank might have been fired, or even worse, lost his pension. These adventures only served to increase Diane's anxiety and her need for control. But the way she expressed her anxiety was giving her husband an excuse to act out. Diane could become very demonstrative and even bossy in her approach. Hank took this as especially emasculating. Diane had a history of being involved with men who were out-of-control such as alcoholics and drug addicts. Her conflict around control was evident in her choice of men. She worked so hard to control their behavior but given the depth of their problems, this was almost impossible.

The evidence was mounting that the couple suffered from an unbalanced conflict around control. They each had control issues prior to meeting, which their collusion served to exacerbate. This begs the question: Where did their individual control conflicts come from? For the answer I constructed and carefully examined their respective genograms.

Genogram

Hank was raised in a poor, single-parent family. His father and mother divorced when he was 10-years old. He has three older siblings all of whom are females. Hank claimed that he was always pushed around by his mother and sisters. While they worried about him getting into trouble, he felt smothered. Hank admitted that his mother and sisters meant well and probably saved him from the streets. But he also felt controlled by them and at times perceived their behavior as emasculating. This was evidence that Hank suffered from an internalized *control versus out-of-control* conflict which was causing him marital problems in real time.

Diane's genogram revealed that she was the middle sibling of four. She had a dominant father and a passive mother. She said that her father was a micromanager and controlled everything from the finances to family vacations. He dictated where his children went to college, which college, and what they should major in. He also would determine when his children dated and with whom. Diane reported that she was the only one in the family to challenge her father and did so on a regular basis. But with every challenge, Diane suffered the wrath of his temper and the negative feedback from her enabling mother and siblings, who supported him out of fear.

Diane reported that she walked on eggshells in her family of origin because she never knew when her father would try to exert his massive control. She was especially disappointed that she had to stand alone against her father. This confirmed my belief that Diane like Hank, had developed a *control versus out-of-control* conflict. Diane grew up in a tightly controlled, fearful environment. But once she left home for college, she took control of her own life and never looked back. She said leaving home was like escaping from prison. While much of her father's control was for the best, it also thwarted Diane's growth and left her with little confidence. While Diane resisted being controlled, she would pay for it with anxiety.

Content Versus Process

In treating Hank and Diane, it was helpful to realize that the couple's "process" was an underlying *control versus out-of-control* conflict and that the primary "content" as presented by the couple was financial. That is, each partner's conflict regarding the need to gain and lose control developed into an external conflict over money. There were struggles in other contexts, such as the couple's struggle over seeking professional help. But the couple's most serious disagreements and subsequent control struggles were about money.

Assessing Jordan and Cheryl: A Sexual Control Struggle (See Figure 5.2)

Initial Contact and Chief Complaint

Cheryl called me on the telephone. While she was pleasant and relatively open about her problem, there seemed to be a hint of embarrassment. She told me that she suffered from inhibited orgasm, claiming that she had never achieved an orgasm in her life, either by her own hand or with a partner. She said that she felt both flawed and frustrated, but that her husband Jordan was especially upset. Apparently, Jordan felt emasculated by his inability to make his wife orgasm. He stopped initiating sex with Cheryl and reported that his sex drive for her had waned—but not yet disappeared. He questioned whether she was attracted to him, but also believed that she was too "uptight" about sex. According to Cheryl, because she has procrastinated about seeking help, she believes that her husband's commitment to treatment was now somewhat tenuous. The couple were in their late 30s and had been married for eight years; they had one small child.

First Session

Jordan presented as frustrated but somewhat empathic about his wife's sexual difficulty. But his perception of the couple's problem was astutely broader than his wife's. Although he did not make the connection between control and her orgasm problem, he did feel that she had a strong need for control in all aspects of their lives. He confirmed that she was an anxious person, but he felt that her need for control had less to do with anxiety and more to do with a strong need

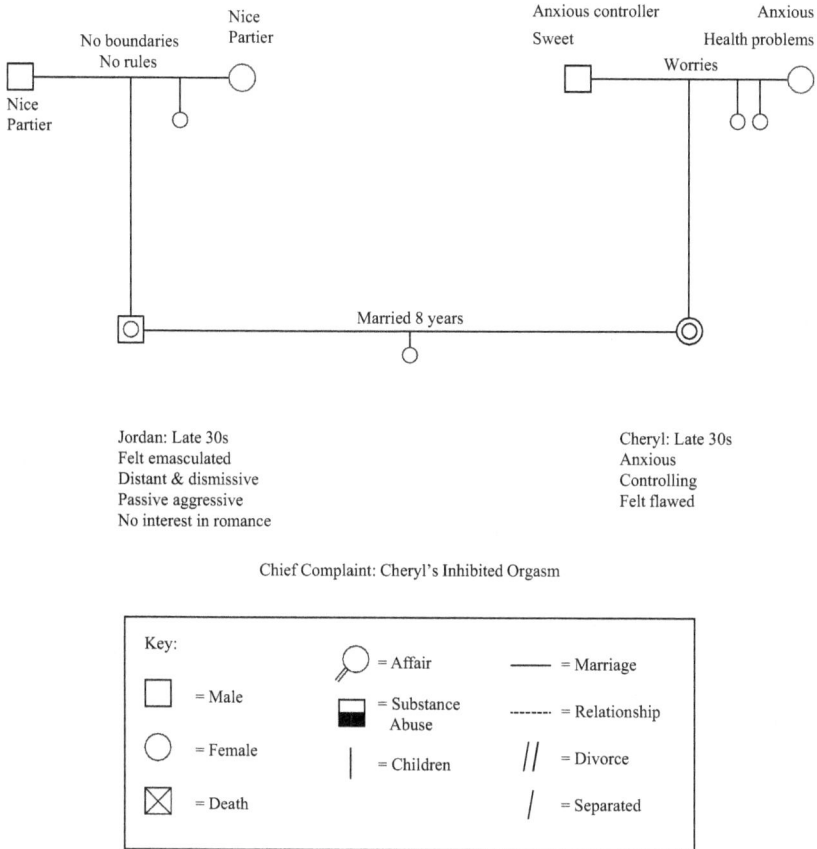

No boundaries
No rules

Nice
Partier

Nice
Partier

Anxious controller
Sweet

Worries

Anxious
Health problems

Married 8 years

Jordan: Late 30s
Felt emasculated
Distant & dismissive
Passive aggressive
No interest in romance

Cheryl: Late 30s
Anxious
Controlling
Felt flawed

Chief Complaint: Cheryl's Inhibited Orgasm

Key:

☐ = Male

○ = Female

⊠ = Death

○ = Affair

■ = Substance Abuse

| = Children

―――― = Marriage

------- = Relationship

// = Divorce

/ = Separated

Figure 5.2   Jordan and Cheryl.

to be the boss. Cheryl admitted that she was controlling and somewhat of a perfectionist, but she thought Jordan was as well. She said that he often fought her decisions and made plenty of his own.

Because the couple presented with a sexual problem, I took a sexual history in the first session and looked for control issues in each partner's pasts. There was no evidence of physical or sexual abuse. Both lost their virginity in high school, and neither were from strict religious backgrounds. Because they were attractive people, they did have extensive dating histories but practiced serial monogamy. Although Cheryl was the symptom-bearer, she was the more affectionate of the two. Jordan did not suffer from any sexual disorders but as mentioned, he had become less sexually interested in Cheryl and more apathetic towards her in general. As she reported in the initial contact, Cheryl has never achieved orgasm. She tried masturbating by hand and with a vibrator but as she would put it: "As I got close, a wall would suddenly come down." She rarely fantasized. Neither reported any paraphilias or fetishes.

When Cheryl was asked to assess Jordan's sexual skills, she was less than enthusiastic. She said there was little foreplay because Jordan likes to go right to intercourse. "He's not a big kisser," she said, "nor is he the romantic type." Indeed, Jordan was not interested in the seduction process which Cheryl preferred. But he countered that it did not matter what he did because nothing would work with Cheryl. Jordan also said on that rare occasion that Cheryl did use a vibrator she would stop it or pull it away before she could reach orgasm. He reiterated that Cheryl cannot seem to tolerate being out of control.

Both partners agreed that they were physically attracted to each other but when I separated the couple to inquire about sexual abuse and affairs, Cheryl admitted that she probably was not as attracted to Jordan as he was to her but added that the disparity is not enough to cause her inhibited orgasm. She claimed that she had this problem with all her ex-boyfriends regardless of their attractiveness, and that two of them broke up with her because of it. Neither she nor Jordan was on any medication, and Cheryl reported no pain during intercourse. Neither partner had any difficulty with oral sex, but Jordan said that Cheryl did not particularly like to receive it.

I believe that Jordan was right about Cheryl's need for control. Orgasm disorders are, for the most part, about an inability to let go. And just as she was about to let go sexually, Cheryl would block orgasm. It is also a sign of control that she did not like oral sex performed on her and that she needed to be on top sexually or in the female superior position to have sex at all. But there were other signs of control as well. Cheryl would block any trips that Jordan wanted to take and usually blamed it on money. She would also limit their socializing with friends. In her work as an elementary school teacher, she admitted that she was part teacher and part disciplinarian.

Cheryl was also right about Jordan, who did what he could to avoid being controlled. To achieve this, he would distance or be passive aggressive. For example, Jordan created his own little world apart from Cheryl. He would buy things without telling her, set up bank accounts in secret, and even socialize without her knowing. He would also emotionally distance and would refuse to kiss her during lovemaking. Often, he would roll his eyes when she asked him for something or "yes" her without ever acting on whatever he agreed to. He even made plans to go back to school without discussing it with her. His excuse was that he did not want her in his business because she would take over. He also refused to work on his foreplay and showed little interest in romancing his wife. Consider the following exchange:

Jordan: I can't do anything without Cheryl sanctioning it. Sometimes I feel like I am in prison and the warden makes all the decisions.

Therapist: But you do seem to fight her control.

Jordan: Yeah, but for the most part I sneak around. Why should I have to do that? I'm not a little kid. I did well enough before I met her.

Cheryl: Actually, you were lost. You had trouble finishing college and you were in debt.

Therapist: You both have something of value to offer but neither of you seem to accept that. Instead, you are fighting each other for control to no avail.

The couple's conflict about control showed itself in that they were repeatedly feeding back into their problem. The more Cheryl exerted control over Jordan the more passive aggressive and secretive he became, thus diluting Cheryl's control. The more elusive Jordan became the more controlling Cheryl felt the need to be. While this dynamic was prominent in the couple's sex life, it was evident in their overall lifestyle as well. To validate that the couple suffered from a *control versus out-of-control* conflict I constructed an extensive genogram on each partner.

Genogram

Cheryl was the oldest of three sisters. She got along with her parents and looked to them for guidance but described both as "worriers." She said that her mother was on anti-anxiety medication and suffered from some serious health problems. She claimed that because he had three daughters, her father was a sweet man but also an "anxious mess." Their worry transformed into a risk aversion and Cheryl grew up finding it more and more difficult to stretch herself and to follow her dreams. Every time she came up with an idea, her parents would warn her about the potential consequences. It was also difficult for her family to relax and have fun. For example, the family rarely went on vacations, but if one were planned, Cheryl reported that it would be canceled at the last minute, for a variety of reasons: medical or transportation issues, or another type of family crisis. Allowing pleasure was too risky.

In tune with a pleasure inhibition and a need for security, it became evident that although Cheryl seemed committed to making her marriage work, she was not very attracted to Jordan. What she did see in him, however, was that he was a kind, solid man who would provide her with the security she craved. The concepts of passion and physical attractiveness took second place to these characteristics.

Cheryl said that her parents were not anti-sex. She also claimed that they were affectionate with each other. But they seemed obsessed about sexually transmitted disease (STDs) and pre-mature pregnancy. As a result, Cheryl said that she was too focused on a potential catastrophe to relax and allow herself to experience sexual pleasure.

Jordan had a younger sister who he was reasonably close with. He described his parents as nice people who enjoyed themselves, almost to a fault. According to Jordan, there was always a party at his house and relatives and friends were constantly in and out. He said that his household was so much fun that it made it difficult for him to leave, but he and his parents agreed he should follow his own path. While Cheryl did not mention this, I believe that another aspect of her attraction to Jordan was his ability to have fun, free of worry.

The downside to Jordan's family of origin was that there were few boundaries and little to no limit-setting. He said that his parents were not involved in his decision-making and rarely offered advice. He said that he had to "go it alone." When he did approach them about something that was bothering him, they were nice but rarely took anything seriously. He said life was a big party. Nevertheless, Jordan claims that he is still close to his family and enjoys being with them. Unlike Cheryl's path, Jordan was much more scattered. He went to three colleges, partied a lot, and repeatedly changed his majors. He only later completed his degree. Cheryl's path was tightly structured, thanks in part to her parents. She completed her bachelor and master's degrees at the same institution and went right into the work world.

It was obvious that Cheryl provided Jordan with the structure he needed, and he tried to provide Cheryl with a love of life. Unfortunately, each partner failed to see the value in the other's approach and a conflict around control developed. Jordan needed structure but freedom as well. Cheryl needed to loosen up but feared the consequences of doing so. Cheryl's sexual inhibition was disturbing, but conquering it was perceived as scary; pleasure had its consequences. Jordan needed a controlling partner, but he felt that her inability to have fun detracted from his.

Content Versus Process

The content in this case cut across a variety of contexts such as travel, socializing, and finances. But the predominant context was Cheryl's sexual inhibition and her chief complaint of achieving orgasm. The process proved to be a *control versus out-of-control* conflict. The longer this conflict remained unbalanced and reinforced by the couple, the more symptomatic they were, and the greater chance that their marriage would continue to deteriorate. The assessment revealed that the case was appropriate for a couples therapist with a sex therapy background.

Assessing the Therapist-Couple Fit

Up until this point the assessment phase has focused primarily on client assessment. But sometimes, the therapist is ill-equipped to treat a particular client. If the therapist detects this early enough, he/she might be able to avoid control struggles. For example, colleagues and supervisees have presented cases to me which they found too difficult to treat for a variety of reasons. A former female supervisee found the husband of a couple to be physically threatening. The couple was ordered by the court to seek counseling because of a domestic violence issue. The supervisee reported that the couple could only be seen later in the evening and that the husband was physically intimidating with a booming voice and several ominous tattoos. He also had a criminal record and had spent time in prison. She believed that he used his size and reputation to intimidate her . . . and it was working. Rather than get into a control struggle with the adamant supervisee I sanctioned the referral. She was then able to make a friendly exit by voluntarily giving up all evening hours.

Older clients, celebrities, or even successful professionals may stir up feelings of inadequacy in some therapists. It is quite easy for powerful clients to challenge a therapist, especially if they sense a lack of confidence on the therapist's part. This is often the case when the clients are therapists themselves. Therapists as clients can be intimidating to some therapists if they make it a habit of challenging their expertise. This is more likely to happen if the treating therapist and the clients follow different therapeutic models. Nevertheless, the therapist must stay in control and think of these challenges as a defense against change. I have never sanctioned a referral based on a supervisee's concern about their intellectual abilities.

In other situations, an inexperienced therapist might feel adventurous and take on a case that was out of his/her area of expertise (DeAngelis, 2018). This decision is in tune with *control versus out-of-control* conflict because it will usually end up with the therapist feeling out-of-control. A colleague took on a couple in which the husband had dissociative disorder but had no idea how to treat it. He thought that if he simply read a book on the topic that would be enough. But this turned out to be a disaster. The client became enraged over some of the interventions that the therapist offered and threatened to sue. The therapist was forced to seek out a supervisor with special expertise in this area.

And finally, a couple may stir up certain feelings in the therapist or a countertransference (Freud, 1910/1957) that he/she is not able to emotionally handle. Freud wrote the following on the concept of countertransference:

> Other innovations in technique relate to the physician himself. We have become aware of the 'counter-transference', which arises in him as a result of the patient's influence on his unconscious feelings, and we are almost inclined to insist that he shall recognize this counter-transference in himself and over-come it.
>
> (pp. 144–145)

For more on countertransference see "Chapter 7. How the Couples Therapist Can Avoid Being Caught in a Control Struggle." But for now, I will offer three brief examples on the subject: A female colleague confessed to me that she had trouble working with a couple in which the wife was pregnant. My colleague was having difficulty getting pregnant herself and felt that the emotional strain on her would adversely impact the couple. She decided to refer the couple rather than attempt to work through her issues with the case.

Another colleague recently lost her mother to cancer and could not bring herself to work with anybody who had a serious illness. She was offered a contract with a cancer treatment facility who agreed to refer her all their patients, but she refused and recommended someone else for the job. And finally, a colleague who had been sexually abused could not bring herself to treat any clients who suffered from sexual problems. She was not inclined to work on this issue and would refer almost immediately.

We know that a "fit" between the couple and the therapist is a key component in successful treatment. The therapist and couple must form a strong alliance (Davis et al., 2019; Friedlander et al., 2018), especially to avoid control struggles. However, most therapists cannot relate to everybody. The art of couples therapy is to join with two people and to treat them equally and objectively. Each must believe that the therapist has their best interests at heart. This is a difficult task to accomplish when partners are fighting, and constantly looking for an edge in their control struggle.

Getting the therapist to side with them against their partner holds great value. I always recommend that the therapist experience as much of life as possible— the more diverse the experiences the better. Travel can help the therapist to relate to couples from different cultures. Connecting with friends and colleagues who can offer different perspectives on life can prove useful. In working with couples, it is not necessary, but helpful if the therapist has been in at least one long-term relationship or marriage. Clients with children may only feel comfortable if the therapist has children.

While a couples therapist might feel discriminated against if a couple rejects him/her, the therapist must keep in mind that most of the time the couple are looking for someone they can relate to. There is no percentage in trying to "sell a couple" on the advantages of seeing you. It will only turn the couple off and it may damage your integrity. Not to mention that it is a surefire way to start a control struggle with a couple. Many years ago, I had the opportunity to gain the trust of several lesbian couples in a nearby city. However, I initially did not know what I was doing. I had great success with gay male couples, but I soon realized that lesbian couples had their own idiosyncrasies. I was totally baffled by the amount of egalitarianism in these couples, and how flexible they could be in shifting roles; this was certainly unlike most of my heterosexual clients (Green, 2014). I soon decided to stop seeing lesbians, read more about them, and to seek a consultation with an experienced lesbian therapist. It was tremendously helpful.

Many believe that therapists—especially couples therapists who are regarded for their ability to balance a couple—like and respect everybody. But this is simply not true (Baker, 2009). Many supervisees have complained to me over the years: "I do not like the husband" or "I cannot stand the wife." Some supervisees have requested that I approve a referral. Indeed, some clients are rude and there is nothing more unpleasant for a couples therapist than having a couple join in arms against him/her. A female supervisee reported that the wife of a couple was verbally abusive to her in treatment. While the supervisee assured me that she was empathic to the wife's plight, the wife continued to vigorously attack her. Apparently, the wife was too afraid to go after her husband for fear he would leave her, so she took her anger out on the therapist. This was not, however, productive because the therapist eventually wanted out of the treatment. When the therapist let on that she was going to refer the couple, the wife insisted she keep the case and a control struggle ensued.

People tend to be attracted to others like themselves, and if you are not anything like your clients it will be harder to join with them. The therapist can try to hide any differences, but clients know what they like, and it would not be unusual for the therapist to inadvertently trigger something in the client that highlights these differences. I always encourage therapists to understand—at the deepest level possible—what has happened in the treatment before they part ways. For example, a supervisee reported that she wanted to refer the husband of a couple and keep the wife for individual therapy. The therapist claimed that the husband was flirtatious and solicitous and that this made her feel uncomfortable. She did not want to tell his wife how she felt but she wanted to refer him under the guise that he could use individual therapy.

Considering the husband's backstory, I concluded that the supervisee was right about him: he did repeatedly cross boundaries. So, my first suggestion was that the therapist ask his wife what she thought about his behavior. But the supervisee refused; she only wanted to stop working with this couple. I then showed her that she was feeding into this man's pathology. She neglected to see that he unconsciously instigated being fired or kicked out of treatment, which was in turn a replication of his mother abandoning him as a child. The supervisee was fascinated but not moved. It took several supervisory sessions, including an analysis of my own need for control, to keep my supervisee on the case.

To keep or to refer an ongoing case can be a complicated issue. But the best way to avoid being in this position is to make as quick an assessment of the case as possible and to make a move as soon as possible. Once the treatment starts it is harder to refer; and if a control struggle is underway, abruptly stopping treatment could end in disastrous consequences for clients and therapist. A couple may feel abandoned and rejected and may file a complaint against the therapist. In the initial contact the therapist must be honest with him/herself. Asking the following questions of him/herself may help:

Do I feel uncomfortable treating the couple?
This is the first question that you should ask yourself and it is a general one. If you answer "yes" to this question you should continue to ask yourself the rest of these questions to arrive at the specific reason for your discomfort. Sometimes you will simply get a gut feeling that you should not take the case, but you should follow it through and arrive at an intellectual reason for your rejection, if possible.

Does the couple scare me?
If you feel threatened in any way you will need to acknowledge this and determine how much of it is real.

Do I have the expertise to help them?
If you do not have the training and experience to treat a particular problem, refer the case to someone who does. Couples therapy is not a research experiment, and on-the-job training could prove dangerous and damaging.

Did I instantly dislike the couple?

I believe that the way a case starts is usually the way a case will end. Therefore, from the initial contact if the client or couple irritate you, you might try to understand it sooner rather than later. Often the couple could be tapping into something from your past making it difficult for you to treat them objectively.

Do I get a sense that there is a mutual commitment to treatment?

Do not get into a control struggle with a couple around their commitment. It would be best to assess this commitment and if you are not comfortable, refer them with no hard feelings. As previously discussed, it is common for one partner to commit while the other will not or will only do so under duress. This needs to be sorted out and if you have an ambivalent partner you might want to first recommend individual therapy for each until the couple can come together and agree to commit to the process.

How many therapists has the couple seen?

It is not uncommon for a couple to make a poor choice of therapist. But some couples make it a habit of jumping from one therapist to the next and in the process using them as scapegoats for their failure to improve. It is as if on an unconscious level, the couple wants their therapists to fail so that they can avoid change.

Will this case end up in the legal system?

If you are shy of the legal process, you can ask your clients if their case has the potential to end up in court. You are at greater risk if the couple is prone to control struggles and is on the verge of divorce. If the couple has young children, there might be an increased probability of legal action over custody. It is also common for those that suffer from addiction to run into legal trouble.

Will I be at risk financially?

To avoid a control struggle around the fee, make certain you have discussed your fee arrangement with the couple and that they are clear about your policy on this matter. This would include not only the price of each session, but how and when you expect to be paid. And do not forget to discuss payment for missed appointments. Too many therapists are concerned about the exchange of money and fail to be clear about what their financial expectations are. If you experience a couple that from the onset fight you about the fee, for whatever reason, it might be best to refer them to someone who charges less.

I have run into control struggles with clients about my billing process. While I am usually paid after each session, I provide couples with receipts or statements once a month. Even though I am clear about this in the initial contact, some couples have requested that I get them out sooner. I hold my ground but try and maintain control over my process. On some occasions a couple may be unrealistic about their ability to afford my treatment. If you do not think a couple can cover your fee it is best to bring this up.

Is this couple being sincere or do they just want to use me in the legal system or otherwise?

In some instances, a couple may not be sincere about seeking treatment but rather want a letter either for legal or other nonclinical purposes. If the therapist misses this, or refuses to provide this reference, a control struggle may ensue. The best way to combat this is to vet the client as carefully as possible. And above all, try and stay away from anything that is beyond your specific level of expertise.

Do I feel that the couple will abide by the rules of treatment?

Aside from potential issues with the fee, you must get a sense that the prospective couple will abide by the terms of the treatment. That is, they will not only pay the fee in a timely fashion but maintain appropriate boundaries and succumb to your setting of limits. This might prevent your clients from giving you hugs and kisses after a session, or buying you presents. These maneuvers may be out of the goodness of the couple's heart, but they may also serve to unbalance the treatment. If you come to believe that setting limits with one or both partners has in of itself become a struggle for control and that no conversation with them will have a positive impact . . . refer. Maybe another couples therapist will fare better.

There is usually no such thing as an easy couple's case. And therapists must take some risks. But if your gut tells you that you cannot be of help then by all means, refer. There is a way to do this without hurting or enraging the couple and it is vital not to get into a control struggle with them over the issue. I usually recommend that the therapist present the referral in a way that suggests he/she cannot help, and that the couple will be wasting their time and money. Sometimes I suggest that a specialist is the better way to go.

Recently a woman called with a host of serious physical problems. While she wanted sex therapy for her and her husband, it immediately occurred to me that their significant health issues and the numerous medications that each were taking was served better by seeing a psychiatrist with a sex therapy background. When listening to her story, I envisioned she or her husband having a health crisis in my office, and I would not know what to do. I also feared I would miss something and cause damage. The woman was somewhat disappointed but understood that I was begging off for the couple's sake.

While the formal assessment phase should be conducted within the first one to two sessions, assessment is an ongoing process (Karson, 2017). That is, while the therapist may be encouraged to draw a preliminary hypothesis from the point of initial contact and through the formal assessment phase, information will continue to flow into the therapeutic process. Therefore, the therapist will need to make continuous adjustments. In some cases, the therapist's hypothesis will be validated and in others, it will merit change. The more astute and experienced the therapist, the less likely he/she will be "completely" off the mark—but it can happen.

Most clinicians have a therapeutic model that they devoutly follow. But it can be a mistake to assume that every client will fit into this model or to take a "one size fits all" approach. According to Karson (2017), this concept may give the clinician the false belief that he/she does not have to take a detailed assessment.

It helps to have a solid theoretical approach to therapy, but the therapist should remain open to incorporating other works into their assessment and treatment phases. For example, if a partner was severely parentified as a child and this was deleteriously impacting his/her need for control in adult relationships, it should not matter whether the therapist practices *Internal Family Systems Therapy* (Schwartz & Sweezy, 2020), *Emotionally Focused Therapy* (Johnson, 2019) or *Master Conflict Therapy* (Betchen & Davidson, 2018). Because the concept of parentification is so closely tied to *Contextual Therapy* (Boszormenyi-Nagy & Spark, 1973), the therapist should consider incorporating some of these principles into the treatment. If a couple is required to remain open in therapy, the couple's therapist should set a proper example of openness.

At the end of the assessment phase, the couple's therapist may want to offer the couple what I refer to as a non-threatening intervention. This could be a comment on their process or content depending on the therapist's discretion. The main objective is to give the couple something useful to think about. I usually refer to it as: "something to chew on between now and the next session." This intervention should not be presented with absolute certainty but should bear some weight; at least enough for the couple to think you understand their plight and have something unique to offer them. Most important, the intervention should be balanced. If you present a couple with an intervention perceived as favorable only to one partner this soon in the treatment, there is a good chance you will never hear from the couple again. If, however, the intervention is appropriately balanced, it could serve to join you with the couple.

For example, Tom and Chelsea presented with Tom's low sexual desire. At the end of the assessment phase—or in this case, at the end of the first session—I told the couple that low sex drive was a common issue and that they were not alone in this struggle. I acknowledged that while it can be perplexing, the good news is that once we figure out what is behind it, there is an exceptionally good chance it can be alleviated. Notice that I did not offer any statistics. One never knows how hard a couple is going to work on their problem and if they fail to improve, I prefer that they do not blame our treatment simply because it did not live up to the cure rates in the literature.

Sometimes I may offer what I call a "preliminary hypothesis" at the end of the assessment. For example, I may tell a couple that I suspect that they have been quietly in battle for some time but that neither recognized it as such. If I am confident that there is a self-help book that captures what the couple are dealing with, I may recommend it, but only if I have already read the book. I also make it clear that there is no pressure to run out and buy the book; the couple can purchase it and read it at their leisure. I do not wish to get into a control struggle over bibliotherapy. Zilbergeld's (1999) popular book, *The New Male Sexuality* is an example of a favorite for those couples with sexual disorders. It is usually perceived as empathic, humorous, practical, and easy to read.

And last, I may offer an in-home exercise that the couple can practice. This might be especially valuable when treating sexual symptoms. H.S. Kaplan (personal communication, October 7, 1987) recommended assigning Sensate Focus exercises to a couple if appropriate. She claimed that these exercises—developed by Masters and Johnson (1966)—are particularly effective in reducing a couple's anxiety, and yet are benign enough not to cause the couple damage if unsuccessful. Both exercises include each partner taking turns caressing the other on both sides of the body. Sensate Focus I, includes a full body caress without the touching of each other's genitals. The more advanced, Sensate Focus II includes genital touching.

The assessment phase is invaluable in the therapeutic process. It allows the therapist to get to know each partner from a deeper perspective and to better see their interactional process at work. It also offers a framework from which to work and allows the therapist to determine the appropriate course of treatment. These elements will be demonstrated in the following section: "Section III. Clinical Treatment."

References

American Psychological Association (2020). *APA dictionary of psychology*. Retrieved August 25, 2021, from https://dictionary.apa.org/symptom-substitution

Angers, L. (2020, August 27). *How sexual fetishism can impact your relationship*. Betterhelp. www.betterhelp.com/advice/intimacy/how-sexual-fetishism-can-impact-your-relationship/

Baker, B. (2009). How to deal with clients you do not like. *Monitor on Psychology, 40*(2). www.apa.org/monito/2009/02/clients

Benson, K. (2020, March 9). *How to find a couple's therapist who can actually help you?* The Gottman Institute. Gottman.com/blog/how-to-find-a-couples-therapist-who-can-help-you/

Betchen, S. (1991). Male masturbation as a vehicle in the pursuer/distance relationship in marriage. *Journal of Sex & Marital Therapy, 17*, 269–278. https://doi.org/10.1080/009262391084042351

Betchen, S. (2005). *Intrusive partners-elusive mates: The pursuer distance in couples therapy*. Routledge.

Betchen, S. (2013a, July 4). The slippery slope of open marriage: The dynamic is more complex than you think. *Psychology Today*. www.psychologytoday.com/us/blog/magnetic-partners/201307/the-slippery-slope-open-marriage

Betchen, S. (2013b, November 29). The role of physical attraction in your relationship: Can you get it if you've never had it? *Psychology Today*. www.psychologytoday.com/bloig/magnetic-partners/201311/the-role-physical-attraction-in-your-relationship

Betchen, S. (2015, September 13). Why we marry people we aren't physically attracted to: The importance of laying a good relational foundation. *Psychology Today*. www.psychologytoday.com/blog/magnetic-partners/201509/why-we-marry-people-we-arent-physically-attracted

Betchen, S. (2019, August 9). How to tell your partner you are not physically attracted: Are you having trouble revealing this to your partner? *Psychology Today*. www.psychologytoday.com/us/blog/magnetic-partners/201908/how-tell-your-partner-you-are-not-physically-attracted

Betchen, S. (2020, June 27). When couples fight about politics: The impact of political disagreement in marriage. *Psychology Today*. www.psychologytoday.com/us/blog/magnetic-partners/202006/when-couples-fight-about-politics

Betchen, S., & Davidson, H. (2018). *Master conflict therapy: A new model for practicing couples and sex therapy*. Routledge.

Birnbaum, G., Kanat-Maymon, Y., Mizrahi, M., & Orr, R. (2018). What fantasies can do to your relationship: The effects of sexual fantasies on couple interactions. *Personality & Social Psychology Bulletin, 45*, 461–476. https://doi.org/10.1177/0146167218789611

Boszormenyi-Nagy, I., & Spark, G. (1973). *Invisible loyalties*. Harper & Row.

Bowen, M. (1978). *Family therapy in clinical practice*. Aronson.

Brown, G. (2021, April). *Overview of paraphilias and paraphilic disorders*. Merck Manual. www.merckmanuals.com/home/mental-health-disorders/sexuality/overview-of-paraphilias-and-paraphilic-disorders

Davis, S., Gonzalez, V., & Sahibzada, S. (2019) Therapeutic Alliance in couple and family therapy. In J. Lebow, A. Chambers, & D. Breunlin (Eds.), *Encyclopedia of couple and family therapy*. Springer, Cham. https://doi.org/10.1007/978-3-319-15877-8_508-1

DeAngelis, T. (2018, May). What should you do if a case is outside your skill set? *Monitor on Psychology, 49*(5). www.apa.org/monitor/2018/05/ce-corner

DeMaria, R., Weeks, G., & Twist, M. (2017). *Focused genograms: Intergenerational assessment of individuals, couples, and families* (2nd ed.). Routledge.

Doherty, W., & Harris, S. (2017). *Helping couples on the brink of divorce*. American Psychological Association.

Freud, S. (1910/1957). The future prospects of psycho-analytic therapy. In J. Strachey (Ed. and Trans.), *The standard edition of the complete psychological works of Sigmund Freud* (Vol. 11, pp. 139–151). Hogarth Press and the Institute of Psycho-analysis.

Friedlander, M.L., Escudero, V., Welmers van de Poll, M.J., & Heatherington, L. (2018). Meta-analysis of the alliance-outcome relation in couples and family therapy. *Psychotherapy, 55*, 367–371. http://doi.org/10/1037/pst0000161

Glass, S. (2021). *The trauma of infidelity*. Reflections by Glass. www.shirleyglass.com/reflect_infidelity.htm

Gonsalves, K. (2020, February 28). *How porn effects relationships: The research & the myths*. Mindbodygreen. www.mindbodygreen.com/0-27470/3-ways-porn-is-affecting-your-relationship-and-what-you-can-do-about-it.html

Gray, D. (2006, November 4). *Setting limits: Understanding boundaries in therapy*. Health Central. www.healthcentral.com/article/setting-limits-understanding-boundaries-in-therapy

Green, R.-J. (2014, December 29). *Interview by Lourdes Garcia-Navarro* [NPR Recording]. Same-sex couples may have more egalitarian relationships, Alliant International University, San Diego, CA.

Gurman, A.S., & Burton, M. (2014). Individual therapy for couples problems: Perspectives and pitfalls. *Journal of Marital & Family Therapy, 40*, 470–483. http://doi.org/10.1111/jmft.12061

Hendrix, H., & Hunt, H.L. (2019). *Getting the love you want: A guide for clinicians* (3rd ed.). St. Martin's Griffin.

Johnson, S. (2019). *The practice of emotionally focused marital therapy: Creating connection* (3rd ed.). Routledge.

Kaplan, H.S. (1995). *The sexual desire disorders: Dysfunction regulation of sexual of sexual motivation*. Brunner/Mazel.

Karson, M. (2017, August 14). There is no real therapy without assessment: Therapy is ongoing assessment and assessment is ongoing case formulation. *Psychology Today*. www.psychologytoday.com/intl/blog/feeling-our-way/201708/there-is-no-real-therapy-without-assessment?amp

Lee, C. (2013). The cross-cultural encounter: Meeting the challenge of culturally competent counseling. In C. Lee (Ed.), *Multicultural issues in counseling: New approaches to diversity* (4th ed., pp. 13–19). American Counseling Association.

Lee, C., & Park, D. (2013). A conceptual framework for counseling across cultures. In C. Lee & D. Park (Eds.), *Multicultural issues in counseling: New approaches to diversity* (4th ed., pp. 3–12). American Counseling Association.

Masters, W., & Johnson, V. (1966). *Human sexual response*. Little, Brown & Company.

Moodley, R., Lenggyell, M., Wu, R., & Gielen, U. (Eds.). (2015). *International counseling: Case studies handbook*. American Counseling Association.

Schwartz, R., & Sweezy, M. (2020). *Internal family systems therapy* (2nd ed.). Guilford.

Sewdayal, Y. (2021, June 7). *Controlling behavior: Signs, causes, and what to do about it*. Supportiv. www.supportiv.com/relationships/controlling-behavior-signs-causes-what-to-do.

Sue, D.W., & Sue, D. (2015). *Counseling the culturally diverse: Theory and practice* (7th ed.). John Wiley & Sons.

Toman, W. (1976). *Family constellation: Its effects on personality and social behavior*. Springer.

Watson, L. (2018, June 29). How to agree on sexual frequency. *Psychology Today*. www.psychologytoday.com/us/blog/married-and-still-doing-it/201806/how-agree-sexual-frequency

Weeks, G., & Fife, S. (2014). *Couples in treatment: Techniques and approaches for effective practice* (3rd ed.). Routledge.

Weeks, G., Odell, M., & Methven, S. (2005). *If only I had known . . . avoiding common mistakes in couples therapy*. Norton.

Zilbergeld, B. (1999). *The new male sexuality* (rev. ed.). Bantam.

Section III

Clinical Treatment

6 Treatment Techniques for Couples With Control Struggles

Transitioning From Assessment to Treatment

Although treatment follows assessment, some clinicians contend that therapy begins with the initial contact. It is, after all, the first step towards addressing long-standing problems. Scheduling the initial appointment in of itself has been found helpful to some. Apparently, the anticipation of treatment can have a positive psychological effect on a client's emotional health. The American Psychological Association (2020) refers to this as the "waiting-list phenomenon."

While many clients are not fortunate enough to feel significant relief prior to treatment, by the end of the assessment phase the couples therapist should at least have enough evidence to substantiate whether a couple is suffering from a conflict around control. Colleagues and supervisees ask me if I reveal the conflict to the couple as soon as I recognize it. The answer is "no." I prefer to build on this information until I am certain it will be effective against a couple's defenses. Some couples may immediately accept that they are in a control struggle and others never will. It is the job of the therapist to have the confidence to be consistent in his/her beliefs; adjustments can be made throughout the treatment process.

Many therapists abandon the core of their therapeutic approaches as soon as they are faced with a couple's formidable defense system; these clinicians scatter to find something else that will bring about immediate results. But the therapist must persevere and accept that it is the couple's job to resist. The couple is in conflict and their unconscious objective is to keep their conflict alive, not to cooperate with the therapist. Allowing a therapist to help resolve their issues runs counter to this objective.

It is a good start if the partners agree on the chief complaint. But many couples feel the need to simplify their problems for fear of what might be discovered. This is a frequent occurrence in sex therapy where most clients prefer their problem to be of a medical nature—something that is not their fault and can be easily treated with a pill or injection. An emotional problem is too vague for many people. It also holds them more accountable and offers no clear path to a cure. Worst of all, it will require them to do some work to change.

If a couple disagrees about the cause of their symptoms, it may be a clear sign of a control struggle. For example, a young man in his 20s insisted that he had

DOI: 10.4324/9781003159100-9

erectile dysfunction (ED), but his girlfriend adamantly disagreed with his assessment. She claimed that he was stressed and was pushing himself to perform. The man's urologist supported the diagnosis of ED and prescribed medication, but it failed to be effective. Under most circumstances, the ED here would be the sole content or the symptom. But after completing my assessment, I thought his girlfriend was right. I surmised the young man was depressed because of a recent death in the family. But rather than grieve his loss, he forced himself to have as much sex as possible to cover his pain. Technically, I saw him as suffering from depression, as well as male hypoactive sexual desire disorder (MHSDD) with secondary ED.

For two weeks the young man insisted on ED exercises. And while I ambivalently prescribed them, it was obvious to me that he was in a control struggle with me, his girlfriend—who soon tired of having failed sex—and his penis. After several failures at intercourse the man finally acquiesced and entered the grieving process; his MHSDD improved as did his ED. The true content that needed to be exposed was a combination of the client's depression, low libido, and associated ED, all of which were enabled by a control struggle.

There are times when a little extra knowledge can alleviate a couple's control struggle and their associated symptoms. For example, a couple in their late 60s reported that they had not had sex for two years and that each had developed a low sexual drive. The husband suffered from significant heart problems and was discouraged from having intercourse by his cardiologist. But after lengthy recovery time, the wife decided that she wanted to have sex again. Refusing to follow suit, the husband claimed that he did not feel turned on anymore and he feared sex would trigger a heart attack. He said he would be satisfied with limited affection and petting; to him this was a better alternative than dying.

With reassurance from the cardiologist and his internist—who he trusted—a book or two on erotic literature, and a prescription for Sensate Focus exercises (Masters & Johnson, 1966), the husband was convinced that it was safe to resume sexual activity with his wife. This was a case of "use it or lose it," which is taken quite seriously by most sex therapists. Health issues sidelined this couple for so long they had almost gotten used to living a sex-free life. I had to get them back in the game, so-to-speak. Interviewing prominent relationship experts, Borrelli (2015) found that sex is considered analogous to a muscle in that without exercise it will atrophy both emotionally and physically. In a study of men aged 55–75, Koskimäki et al. (2008) found that males who have intercourse at least once per week were less likely to develop ED than those less active.

Fortunately, most couples who present to me with sexual difficulty have already been evaluated by a gynecologist or urologist. Those that merit medication for significant anxiety or depression have usually received treatment by a psychiatrist. This is both good and bad. The positive aspect of this is that the client is usually cleared of any organic issues and is on the appropriate medication. This way I can just focus on the therapy. The negative aspect is that in their zeal to help patients, physicians often medicate too quickly or unnecessarily. For example, prescribing ED medication to any man who claims to have erectile disorder may coverup underlying issues such as an incompatible relationship or a severe control struggle. In this case, while the ED symptom might improve, another symptom may take its place and in a different context (APA, 2020). This supports the concept that therapist and physician should work together to provide optimal care for clients (McDaniel & deGruy, 2014).

Treatment Objectives and Process

To treat control struggles using MCT, the couples therapist must strive to meet six major therapeutic objectives to help partners to: (1) realize that they are victims of an internal master conflict over the need for control, which is the source of their symptoms; (2) accept the pervasiveness and potency of their internal conflict; (3) recognize that they share the same conflict; (4) determine the origin of their respective internal conflicts; (5) integrate both sides of their shared control conflict in a way that is both functional and comfortable for each; and (6) differentiate enough to break their control struggle and to alleviate any associated symptoms, nonsexual or sexual.

The objectives are met by a 5-step treatment process: *Step 1. Exposing the couple's control struggle*; *Step 2. Exposing the couple's conflict with control*; *Step 3. Broadening the context of the conflict; Step 4. Examining each partner's family of origin*; and *Step 5. Integrating internal conflict and increasing differentiation* (Betchen & Davidson, 2018, pp. 108–111). Each step is explained and illustrated using six diverse clinical cases, three with nonsexual symptoms and three with sexual symptoms. In using MCT, the couples therapist acts like both an investigator and litigator, gathering evidence and persistently challenging each partner's defenses to reveal information useful to the couple. Gentle but firm confrontation is used to help shift each partner from past to present and back again, illustrating the connection between the two and how the concept of control plays a role.

Couple Exercises

Many therapists rely heavily on exercises to help a couple alleviate their symptoms, nonsexual and sexual. Some place high value on couple communication exercises (Gottman & Silver, 2015). Those who practice the integration of couples and sex therapy employ basic sex therapy exercises (McCarthy & McCarthy, 2013), meditation and the integration of somatic interventions (Fox, 2020), as well as mindfulness techniques (Brotto, 2018). There are, however, those that place less value on exercises and more on the differentiation process in couple's work (Schnarch, 2009).

Because MCT is skewed towards the psychodynamic end of the therapeutic continuum, treatment is primarily insight-focused. That is, exposing a couple's unconscious master conflict, helping them to determine its origin, and aiding them in balancing their conflict, are key. Although general couple exercises or homework such as prescribing certain communication techniques or recommending date nights are almost never prescribed in this approach, traditional sex therapy exercises are still considered useful if tactfully integrated into ongoing psychodynamic work. For example, Sensate Focus I and II exercises (Master & Johnson, 1966) would be recommended to couples who seem anxious about general and sexual intimacy. These are still found useful to help these partners stay in the moment (Weiner & Avery-Clark, 2014; Avery-Clark & Weiner, 2018). I also find them to be a great source of foreplay for couples who have difficulty in this area.

Dilator treatment (Masters & Johnson, 1970) as part of a multidisciplinary program may also be integrated into treatment for GPPPD, especially for what was once referred to as vaginismus (Fertel et al., 2020). Dilators are used in a way that is comfortable for the partner, considering the client's emotional state, sexual developmental stage, tolerance level, and values. For example, some women have never masturbated and feel uncomfortable touching themselves; they prefer that their partner insert the dilators. Others, however, do not trust someone else with this task and prefer to insert the dilators themselves. Many of these women have specifically reported concerns about someone else moving too fast or injuring them during the exercise.

Some women are anxious and require more time to progress through the different dilators which range in size from small to large and are to be used in that graded order. A woman I treated would always repeat the previous exercise with the smaller dilator before she would move on to the next, larger one. For example, just before inserting the second dilator she would insert the first one as a prepping exercise. Before inserting the third dilator she would insert the first and second ones. And just before she would insert the fourth dilator, she would insert the first, second, and third in that order. This ritual was quite effective in reducing her anxiety and prepping her vaginal muscles for easier penetration.

The stop-start exercise (Semans, 1956) is used to treat men with premature ejaculation (PE) (Betchen & Gambescia, 2020). This exercise helps men to gradually learn to control the point just before they ejaculate (Masters & Johnson, 1970). In treating female orgasmic disorder, McCabe et al. (2020) reported the benefits of sanctioning sexual fantasy and increasing comfort with one's own body. In some cases, I may even prescribe the reading of a book on erotic literature or one that helps women to explore their bodies such as Mintz's (2018) *Becoming Cliterate* or Nagoski's (2021) *Come as You Are*.

Before any exercises are offered each partner is asked whether the ones prescribed might offend them from a cultural or religious perspective. For some, certain exercises will remind them of prior traumatic experiences and cause harm. No exercises should be assigned until the couple and therapist mutually agree on the type of exercise and the timing of the assignment. A female client with a history of sexual assault told me that a previous therapist moved too fast with dilator treatment and the client felt as if she were being "re-raped."

The couples therapist must be aware, however, how couples use exercises to gain a sense of control over the therapeutic process. Couples may try to take over by immediately insisting on assigned exercises. I tend to see this more often when a couple present with a sexual disorder, but it can happen with nonsexual symptoms. For example, I am usually asked by the couple to assign homework or to tell them what they should work on in between sessions. As mentioned, some couples request this before I have completed my evaluation. While a couple may be sincere in these requests, others are trying to avoid thinking about their problem. They prefer not to look too deeply into it for fear that they may reveal or discover something unpleasant. Simply put, some want a quick fix. My response is usually polite but firm: "I want the same outcome as you say you do but we may have a different way of achieving it. You can trust that if I think exercises or homework will help, I will consider them." This gives the couple the message that I am on their side, but I am the one in charge.

It is almost routine for couples to ask for exercises if they present with a sexual symptom. Many have researched their disorder on the Internet and have found that most of these disorders are treated with exercises. As I have said before, I am not averse to integrating exercises into my approach, but not before I have completed a detailed evaluation. I also carefully plan if, and when these exercises should be employed. Because this model contends that an underlying conflict is responsible for the couple's symptom, assigning exercises too soon might be sabotaged by the internal conflict, resulting in a setback for the couple. H.S. Kaplan (personal communication, October 7, 1987) suggested that if the couple insist on exercises, it would be fine for the therapist to assign Sensate Focus homework. I have found this to be a good way to avoid an immediate control struggle with a couple and give the therapist time to join with them.

It is common in sex therapy for the non-symptomatic partner to refuse treatment on the notion that it is the other's fault. If the symptom bearer has procrastinated in seeking help the non-symptom bearer inherits an excuse to take this stance; it is a convenient way to avoid taking any responsibility for the couple's symptom. My response to this is: "I know that your partner's procrastination has frustrated you. But in relationships, if one partner has a problem, both do. And I believe you will be an asset to the treatment process."

Another control tactic is for the couple to collude in sabotaging the treatment by not following directions suggested by the therapist. For example, Sensate Focus I exercise does not entail genital caressing, but some partners include this rather than wait to be prescribed Sensate Focus II, which does. Others disagree on the instructions given by the therapist and proceed to fight about it rather than complete it. Still others practice their exercises so sporadically that they are rendered ineffective. The first time this happens I simply reassign the exercise. But if it happens again, I will respectfully point out: "You both might be unconsciously trying to take control of the treatment in a way that will be counterproductive. And I want to help you reach your goals."

The following six cases: three couples with nonsexual symptoms and three with sexual symptoms, are presented as they progress through my 5-stage treatment process. The couples presented are a diverse group that, in my opinion, represents the pervasiveness of control struggles in couples. And while there are many other symptoms caused by control struggles, I have chosen those that I have found most likely to produce this type of gridlock in couples.

Ray and Joan: Nonsexual Symptom— Procrastination (See Figure 6.1)

Joan, a physical therapist, demanded that Ray, an accountant, attend sessions with her because he is delaying marriage. The couple have been dating exclusively for eight years and Ray has yet to propose. Joan wants to have children and she is 35-years old; Ray is 40. Ray claims to want the same thing but he never follows through. Joan has thought of ending the relationship and moving on with her life, but she feels scared and helpless. She is also used to being taken care of. In this control struggle, Joan is using relentless pursuit and threats to end the relationship to gain control; Ray is using avoidance and procrastination to escape being controlled.

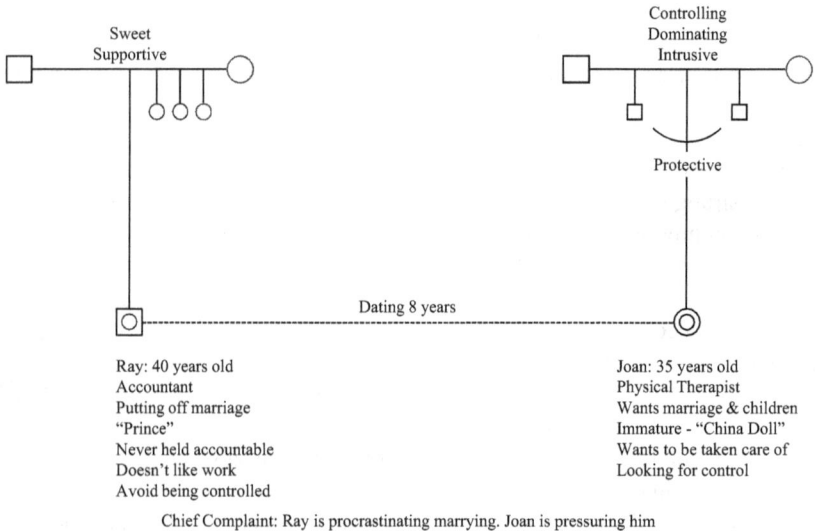

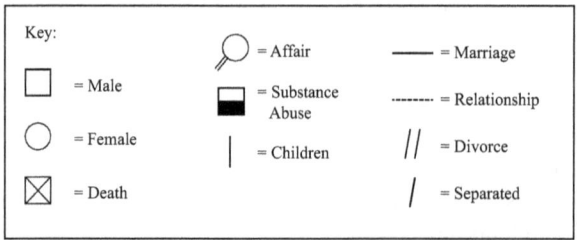

Figure 6.1   Ray and Joan.

Step 1. Exposing the Couple's Control Struggle

In this step, I help the couple uncover their process or their struggle for control in the relationship. In doing so, the first thing I look for is whether partners are giving each other what they want, or whether they are in a standoff. The longer a couple is entrenched in their struggle for control, the more rigid the struggle and the more symptomatic the relationship. Joan and Ray are a good example of this.

Joan: Throughout our dating, Ray told me that he wanted to marry and have children. But I think he lied.

Ray: I didn't lie. I told you I'd like to marry and have kids, but I never gave you a timeline.

Joan: Well, my body has a timeline.

Ray: I can't help that. I just don't feel ready.

Joan: Be honest with me. If you've changed your mind, say so.

Ray: I still want to marry and have kids.

Joan: Well, I thought we could get married this Christmas.

Ray: Maybe we can.

Joan: What does "maybe" mean?

Ray: Maybe means maybe.

Joan: But you have been saying "maybe," "possibly," and "we'll see," for years now and the only thing that is changing is my age.

Ray: (Angrily) That's not true. I think my blood pressure has been steadily rising because of you.

Therapist: It seems as if you two are in a standoff. You both seem to know what the other wants but will not give in. Joan, you want to marry and start a family and Ray, you seem to want to be left alone to contemplate.

Ray: I'm not saying no. I'm just not ready.

Therapist: Yes, I know. But at some point—and I think you may be there—being noncommittal is euphemistic for "no."

Ray: I don't have a definitive answer right now.

Therapist: I'm not trying to pressure you into an answer. And I doubt I could if I tried. My point is that you're locked in, and this could go on indefinitely.

Joan: He won't even give you a straight answer.

Therapist: Yes, but I don't always need a straight answer to decide what I would do in certain situations . . . you seem to. And you relentlessly pursue Ray even though he has made it clear that he's not ready to give you a clear and direct answer. In a sense, you seem just as stuck as he is.

Ray appears to be in control because he will not honor Joan's request to marry and start a family. He does his best to dodge her and instead of being direct, he uses vague words like "maybe" or "possibly" to pacify her. But Joan will not give up. She is obsessed with wearing Ray down. In her pursuit, she torments him and rejects his vagueness. This process has been going on far too long and clearly qualifies as a forbidding control struggle. The therapist reveals this to the couple and points out that they will continue to suffer unless this standoff is resolved. Once the couple accept that control is an issue in their relationship, they are then encouraged to examine the conflict associated with it.

Step 2. Exposing the Couple's Conflict With Control

In this section, partners are encouraged to accept that there are two sides in each of them that are operating at cross purposes with regards to gaining and maintaining control. One effective and efficient way to spot a couple's conflict around control is to look for and highlight any verbal or behavioral contradictions demonstrated by either partner. Specifically, is each partner doing what is needed to achieve their stated objectives, or is he/she sabotaging these objectives? Consider the following example:

Joan: Ray is in control as usual. I can't marry or have children without him.

Therapist: Why can't you?

Joan: What do you mean?

Therapist: Well, how bad do you want to be married and have children?

Joan: Bad. That's what I've been saying all along.

Therapist: Well, it just seems that you perceive Ray as having all the control. But you don't seem to be taking any. Instead, you give it to him. Maybe you're in conflict about having control: you would like some control over your life but do not want to do what it takes to get it. So, you remain stuck and out-of-control.

Ray: I've told her that she can always break up with me.

Therapist: That's a rather cavalier thing to say to a woman who you know will not leave you.

Ray: Well, I don't feel as if I have all the control here.

Therapist: I agree with you. I think that this isn't a healthy situation for either of you. You said that your physical health is suffering. Nevertheless, you cannot seem to make a definitive move even though Joan is apparently torturing you. You may want control—you want to decide if, and when you want to marry and have children—but Joan will not let you have your way. Sounds like you are allowing her to have control over your blood pressure.

Now that the conflict is exposed, the therapist can revisit it at any time. But the therapist is to stick with it no matter what context the struggle shifts to.

This is especially important to show the couple the pervasiveness of their shared conflict.

Step 3. Broadening the Context of the Conflict

Couples often make the mistake of focusing primarily on the symptoms they are experiencing. While this is understandable, internal conflicts do not operate monolithically. That is, their influence is often more pervasive. Couples are almost flabbergasted when I show them the connection between, for example, their internal conflict and other areas of their lives beyond their presented symptom. I call this broadening the couple's context. This technique helps to stop the blame game, joins the couple, and enhances mutual empathy. What follows is a demonstration of broadening the context of Joan and Ray's presented problem utilizing their internal conflict about control:

Therapist: How's work going, Ray? You are an accountant at a firm right?

Joan: Oh, this is a good one. He's fighting with his boss every day.

Therapist: Really?

Ray: He's a jerk. Well, he's not really a jerk but some of the things he wants me to do are unnecessary.

Therapist: Like what?

Ray: He just wants me to be more detailed with my paperwork, and to bill more hours. The usual firm demands.

Therapist: And . . . ?

Joan: Ray wants to do what he wants to do. He's in a big accounting firm, but he has no interest in following orders. One of these days he's going to be fired. I try talking to him, but he won't listen. Instead of working with his boss to move up in his firm, he battles him. I can help Ray, but it doesn't seem to matter to him.

Therapist: So, the control issue is operating at work as well?

Joan: I never thought of it that way, but yes.

Therapist: How do you see it, Ray?

Ray: I just think my boss is a petty micromanager. Why don't we talk about Joan's inability to get a promotion? She's been deserving of one for years, but her bosses keep promoting over her.

Therapist: So, just as she pursues you to marry her, she pursues her bosses to promote her, and she fails at both.

Ray: Very funny.

Therapist: I wasn't trying to be funny.

Joan: It sounds as if you are saying that Ray and I have the same problem with control, and that it's had a general effect on our lives.

Therapist: Yes, that's exactly what I'm getting at; and the proof is that each of you have had it well before you have even met.

Both Ray and Joan would like to have more control at work, but because each are in conflict, neither seem to know how to get it. Ray is potentially sabotaging his career and Joan allows her boss to take advantage of her. If Ray cooperated with his boss, he would no doubt fare better in his career and ultimately have more control over his work world. And Joan wants a promotion, but she overworks and tolerates being repeatedly passed over. In the brief exchange I tried to show each partner the pervasiveness of their shared internal conflict and its relationship to their control struggle. Both partners were surprised by my interpretation.

Step 4. Examining Each Partner's Family of Origin

In this section, we examine both Ray and Joan's respective families of origin to determine the underlying cause of their shared control struggle. Showing the couple that they have a history of control struggles that emanate from their pasts helps to validate the control theory and serves to join them.

Ray is the oldest of four siblings; he has three sisters. He described his parents as sweet, supportive people. Ray admittedly said that he was the "prince" of the family. Rarely was he criticized by family members or held accountable for his behavior. He dropped out of college twice only to go back and finish the third time around. Ray was a smart man, but he joined a fraternity and spent most of his college years admittedly half-drunk. He said he rarely went to class in his first two tries, but finally realized that he had no other life options. Oddly, his parents rarely interfered in Ray's escapades. All Ray could remember is his father making an off-handed remark that college was not for everyone.

Ray said that before meeting Joan, he saw himself as a lifelong bachelor. He said that he was in command of his life, and once he began to earn good money, he saw no need to commit to anybody; he has no history of long-term relationships. Ray said the great thing about being single was that at any time he could get a pizza, put his feet up and put on a football game without anybody bothering him. He claimed that Joan pressured him to marry, and he decided to go along for the ride. He said that it might be fun to have sons to play ball with but that he could live happily without children. He did admit to telling tell Joan that he would have children if she wanted them badly enough.

If Ray's family was "hands off," Joan's was "hands on." Her parents were completely dominating, but in a nice way. She said she knew that they cared about her, but they insisted on making all the major decisions in her life. Joan's parents chose the college she attended as well as her major. Joan has an older and a younger brother both of whom were protective of her. Joan said that she felt safe but immature—like a "china doll." She wanted to be independent, but she also enjoyed the safety and security that her parents and siblings provided.

While it may look like Ray and Joan are opposites, they are similar in perhaps the most important way: they both have a conflict about being in control. Joan cherished independence and admired this trait in others, especially in Ray. But she wanted to be taken care of and was willing to sacrifice control for it. Ray was treated as if he were special by his parents and three doting sisters. He admitted that he was enabled. Rarely if ever was his judgement questioned or held accountable. He also grew up free of any responsibilities. Ray claimed that he never cleaned a dish or took out the trash while growing up; he never even held a job until he became a full-time accountant.

No one told Ray what to do and he was not going to let Joan start. Whether it be his wife or boss, Ray was not interested in being lectured. He tried to live as free of rules as possible. While one part of Ray wanted complete control perhaps more than most, he was lonely and admitted feeling a little "weird" that he did not have a steady woman in his life. While he tried to trade off some control to be more connected, in meeting Joan he got more than he bargained for. Joan did give Ray as much freedom as she could tolerate, and is far from a dictator, but in this one context she has doggishly tried to hold Ray accountable and responsible for initially telling her that he would marry and have children. The following scene illustrates how the therapist helped the couple to connect their backgrounds and their control struggle:

Therapist: Wow Ray, it sounds like you were free to do whatever you wanted in your family of origin. I bet your parents didn't even check your report card when you were a kid.

Ray: Nope.

Therapist: Does the IRS even bother you to pay taxes?

Ray: (Chuckles)

Therapist: So, you committed to Joan, sort of, and you now must feel like you're in prison. It must be hard for a guy who was never asked to take any responsibility, to take on a wife and children. You were never trained for this moment.

Ray: I'll handle it when I'm ready.

Therapist: I'm not so sure. Your parents seemed like nice people, but they might have been too nice. Perhaps they didn't prepare you for how tough the world can be.

Ray: They were great people.

Therapist: Sure . . . but being nice is not what parenting is all about. Parents sometimes have to say things to their kids that the kids don't want to hear. This can prepare them for the real world where they won't be treated so gingerly. I suspect you're having trouble adjusting.

Ray: I'm not having trouble.

Therapist: Well, let's see. You're having trouble with your girlfriend and your boss. That means that you're having trouble adjusting to both your professional and personal lives. What else is there?

Ray: And you think this is because my parents were too nice to me?

Therapist: I suspect so.

Ray: Well, how do you explain my commitment to Joan?

Therapist: How do you explain it?

Ray: I don't know.

Therapist: So, you want me to figure this out for you? You want me to do the work for you?

Ray: No, but I really don't know how to explain it. Please.

Therapist: I think you were lonely and feeling odd about your life. Sometimes we need guidance to feel as if we matter. I think you missed that in your parents. I think you longed for a little structure, so you gave in and entered a relationship with Joan. But you still don't want to be told what to do—something we all must deal with in a relationship. I think you're in conflict.

Ray: Maybe I did miss some of that. But marriage and kids are more than a little responsibility.

Therapist: Agreed.

Joan: Why didn't you tell me you were scared? I would've moved on and founds somebody else.

Therapist: Maybe you would have Joan. But from the looks of your family of origin, you've been so completely controlled I cannot help but think you needed a controlling man like Ray in your life. Life might have been too scary for you without that. And you've admitted that there was safety and security in giving up control to someone else. How does it feel now? Do you feel safe and secure?

Joan: Absolutely not. Now I want some control. Are you saying that my parents helped to inhibit my growth and independence?

Therapist: Something like that. You have internalized a conflict around having control which emanates from your childhood.

You can see how the therapist links the present to each partner's past and pays special attention to the concept of control and any potential conflict that might surround it. If Ray seemed more controlling than Joan, keep in mind that people unconsciously not only choose partners with the same conflict, but a conflict with the same level of intensity. In this case, Joan is just as dug into her position as Ray is to his; their conflicts are of equal strength. This is what makes for an especially challenging control struggle.

Step 5. Integrating Internal Conflict and Increasing Differentiation

As mentioned in "Chapter 1. Introduction: Control and Conflict," to break a control struggle each partner must give up something important to them in their respective families of origin that enables a need to be out-of-control. It is a delicate balance that is quite challenging given that almost every individual has a strong tendency to want it all—to avoid loss at all costs. Couples spend years in treatment trying to have it both ways. At times, it seems as if they are waiting for a miracle. In the MCT approach, it becomes incumbent upon the couples therapist to help each partner to integrate the two seemingly opposite parts of themselves with regards to control; this is the way to help a couple balance or regain balance of their conflict, and to alleviate any associated symptoms.

The good news is that when both sides of conflict are made conscious to each partner, they will benefit greatly from this insight. But they must then bring their newfound information to the couple interaction and negotiate a compromise on control. It is up to each partner to grapple with their own contribution to the control struggle. The therapist must stay neutral and refrain from judging either partner. Once the control struggle is out in the open the couple will continue to show signs of it in treatment that the therapist can easily interpret. The therapist almost never has to abandon his/her approach to treatment. The job now is to repeatedly interpret for the couple—across whatever contexts they present—the way in which these contexts are linked to their conflict around control. Waelder (1960) claimed that the therapist's job is "to open the areas of conflict widely and clearly, with a view to discovering possible unconscious elements, ultimately to help the patient 'to make peace with himself'" (p. 220). The following is an example of how Joan and Ray fared in this process:

Joan: I think what you're saying is that Ray and I are more alike than we think.

Therapist: Yes, you both seem to have the same conflict.

Joan: We both want to be in control?

Therapist: Yes, but it is a bit more complicated than that. Think conflict.

Joan: You mean we both need control, but we also have a need to be out-of-control?

Therapist: That's it.

Ray: I know you've explained this and where it comes from, but it's just too weird for me. Why would anyone want to give up control? Even if we got mixed messages about control from our parents why would either of us want to live by those messages?

Therapist: That's a great question Ray. I understand this is counterintuitive for the both of you, but most couples react the same way when I expose this. Having control has been great for you in so many ways. Would you agree?

Ray: I guess.

Therapist: Nobody told you what to do. You were the "golden boy."

Joan: That's for sure.

Therapist: Ray?

Ray: Yeah, that's true.

Therapist: Okay . . . so most of us never had that experience. Some of us were hounded by our parents to get good grades and to do chores; others rarely saw their parents. But your parents were present and loving, but they were also "hands off." You were the chosen one. You were even spoiled by your sisters.

Ray: You could say that.

Therapist: So, you were in complete control over your own life; you made major decisions without interference. Can you imagine the average child dictating to their parents where and when they will go to college? But you could.

Ray: Okay that's a case for why I want control, but what's the case for not wanting it?

Joan: Everybody needs some structure.

Ray: I was doing fine on my own.

Therapist: If that's true, why have you been with Joan all this time?

Joan: He says he was doing fine but he lived like a hermit in a rundown apartment. And he had no friends. He had a pathetic life.

Therapist: Maybe, but he was in control. The only person he had to answer to was his boss, and he even gave him a hard time.

Ray: So, I still don't get how being with Joan demonstrates a desire to give up control.

Therapist: Whenever we commit to someone or something, we give up something to get something. How is it going with Joan?

Ray: If it were great, I wouldn't be here.

Therapist: Right . . . and it's not great because you still want the same amount of control that you've always had. But you can't pull this off. Joan isn't your mother or your father. She wants some control over you and her life as well.

Ray: (Chuckles) Can't you just talk her out of this.

Therapist: That's not my job.

Ray: So, I must give up some control to Joan?

Therapist: Just some of it, not all.

Joan: I don't want that much anyway. I only want what any woman wants.

Therapist: Joan, how do you see your conflict operating?

Joan: I now see that I'm with Ray because I was used to being taken care of by controlling parents. But I can't take being controlled this much.

Therapist: Right . . . but you sacrificed your independence to be cared for.

Joan: Well, I can't do that anymore.

Therapist: I'm not suggesting either of you made a poor choice of partner. I'm suggesting that your mutual conflict unconsciously selected you for one another. And that there needs to be an adjustment made for your relationship to deepen and thrive. That adjustment will entail that each of you give up some control to get more of it. This way your relationship won't be at risk and your symptoms will most likely dissipate.

Ray: Do we just negotiate the amount of control each of us should take? Joan wants two big things: marriage and children. How can I negotiate that?

Therapist: You might not be able to, but you must acknowledge something that has been difficult for you: that your parents needed to set better limits with you. You must accept the fact that they have helped you to become somewhat averse to responsibility. If you can take more of it, then you might reach a compromise.

Joan: Geez, we are only talking about getting married and having children. I'm not asking you to amputate your leg. Everybody else in America is doing it, why can't you?

Therapist: Ray, you did say that you would like to marry and have kids. Do you ever think about what it would be like to have a child?

Ray: I said this before. I do sometimes think about the prospects of having a catch with my son.

Therapist: That sounds enjoyable to you?

Ray: Yeah, I think that would be fun. I never had a catch with my dad.

Joan: Girls can catch too.

Therapist: So, Ray, to maintain control and avoid being responsible you give up the chance to have a catch with your child? Do you like that deal?

Ray: I never thought of it that way.

Therapist: I know this is hard Ray, but if you want a child you will have to give up being a prince: the golden child.

Ray: (Chuckles).

Therapist: And Joan . . . you blame Ray for controlling you, but you have a history of giving control away for the sake of being cared for. Does that seem like a good deal to you?

Joan: It doesn't when you put it that way. I guess you are saying I need to learn to take care of myself.

Therapist: Sounds about right.

Ray and Joan did well in this most difficult step. They were each brave enough to face the past and to understand how it impacts the present. Specifically, they came to see how each was in conflict about control and what it was costing them as individuals and as a couple. They realized that neither had to completely over-haul their personalities or to choose one part of themselves over the other. Joan did not have to choose safety over independent control and Ray did not have to choose control over a family. But each had to pay a price to integrate these parts. In the next case we will see how to apply this approach with a couple suffering from a different, yet common nonsexual symptom.

Deshawn and Shanice: Nonsexual Symptom— Domestic Chores/Division of Labor (See Figure 6.2)

Deshawn and Shanice are a Black couple. Deshawn was previously married with three children and the couple have two together; all five children reside with Deshawn and Shanice. Deshawn is 44 years-old and Shanice is 36. They have been married for seven years. Shanice is a human resource executive at a large company and Deshawn is head of maintenance at a high school.

Shanice reports that Deshawn acts like a "lazy child." She said he hangs out with his single friends at night clubs and rarely if ever helps with chores around the house. Deshawn thinks that Shanice should be handling domestic chores; he believes that they are a woman's domain. He sees his wife as a nag and wants her to stop bothering him. He said that he is the "man of the house" and finds it emasculating that she hounds him. Shanice counters that she already has five children and does not need another one. She said that she only treats Deshawn like a child because he acts like one.

Deshawn admits that he both hides from and lies to his wife. He is avoidant, dismissive, and passive aggressive in his efforts to escape her. Shanice claims that she cannot reason with Deshawn because he only sees things from his per-spective. She left him once for a few months but returned after he promised he would help her out; but he did not keep his word. Shanice claimed that moving out was traumatic and that she would rather try and work things out rather than leave again. But she employs blaming, bullying, and uses verbal threats to try to control Deshawn. She is again threatening to leave him if he will not do his part in the marriage.

Step 1. Exposing the Couple's Control Struggle

Shanice is a modern woman with a time-consuming career. She claims to need more control of her world and feels that she can only get it with Deshawn's help. However, Deshawn has never given any indication that he was interested in domestic work. He took his children in after his first wife died of a drug overdose, but he rarely spends any time with them. Shanice claimed that he was simply looking for a woman to take on his burden. Deshawn denied this but contradicted himself when he claimed that he wants Shanice to leave him alone and take care of all the family's domestic responsibilities herself. Deshawn is

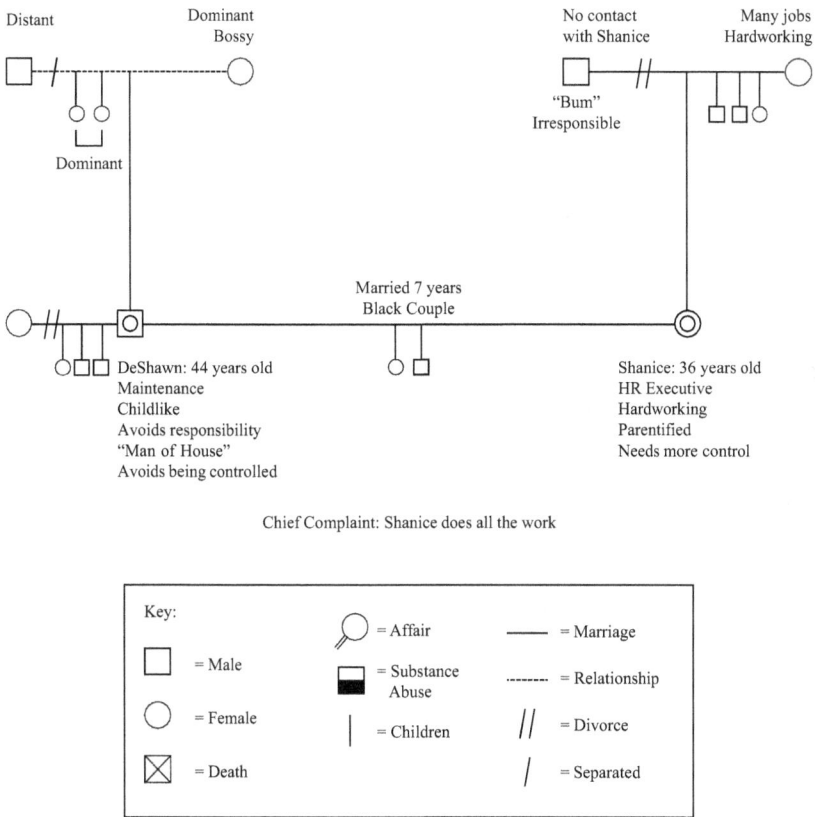

Key:

☐	= Male	⚲	= Affair	———	= Marriage
○	= Female	▭	= Substance Abuse	-------	= Relationship
⊠	= Death	│	= Children	//	= Divorce
				/	= Separated

Figure 6.2   Deshawn and Shanice.

fighting off Shanice's pursuit in a desperate effort to prevent her from controlling him. The following scenario demonstrates how to label and expose the couple's fruitless control struggle:

Shanice: I didn't come back for this. I have five children to take care of and Deshawn is my sixth. He just hangs with his friends and does more for them than he does for me and our family.

Deshawn: She's always picking on me. I'm a man. I don't want to hear all that stuff from her.

Shanice: You think I like picking on you? I hate being a nag, but you turned me into one. You think I'm your mother, but I'm not going to take care of everything for you.

Deshawn: You're not my mother.

Therapist: So, your mother took care of all the chores?

Deshawn: I guess.

Therapist: I assume your mother is up in age. Maybe she's old school. But you've married a modern woman with a career.

Deshawn: My mom worked: she cleaned houses all day and then took care of us.

Shanice: But she was a single mother.

Therapist: Didn't you help her with the chores Deshawn?

Deshawn: Nah, my sisters did.

Shanice: He was spoiled.

Therapist: Maybe, but it now seems that you are trying to train him to be someone different. Wasn't he like this when you met him?

Shanice: But he's worse now.

Therapist: Well, it might look that way, but he now has more responsibility.

Shanice: So, you think he is what he is, and that's it?

Therapist: No, not necessarily. But you and Deshawn seem to be in a standoff that you can't seem to negotiate your way out of. It's not my job to judge, but I can tell you there will be no winner . . . just two losers, unless you stop fighting one another and get on the same page.

Fortunately, the couple was open enough to consider my conflict approach. I believe this had much to do with the fact that despite being at odds, they both wanted to save their marriage. In the next section I address the concept of control with them.

Step 2. Exposing the Couple's Conflict With Control

Shanice wants Deshawn to contribute to household duties, which in this case is like asking him to be more like her. This way Deshawn can help her to control her environment, which at times is overwhelming. She is a mother, wife, and has a demanding career. The problem is that the more Shanice pressures Deshawn, the more he resists her. The more he resists, the more she goes after him. But in the end, neither get much control over their lives. In the following scene the couple is made aware of this contradiction:

Therapist: Shanice, do you think pursuing Deshawn the way you do is working?

Shanice: Obviously not . . . but I don't think anything will work with Deshawn. He's a little boy.

Deshawn: (Angrily) That's what I'm talking about: she disrespects me.

Therapist: I know you're insulted by that comment Deshawn. But do you think your reaction is helping?

Deshawn: Nothing will help.

Therapist: That might be a convenient excuse to avoid helping her. You seem to see her as a boss—as if she is in control.

Deshawn: She "is" the boss.

Therapist: A boss that you don't listen to. Shanice, do you feel in control?

Shanice: Hell no. I feel more out-of-control than ever.

Therapist: I would suggest that you both are in control. Shanice you are in charge. The children take their orders from you and you make the family go. Deshawn, you too are in control because you dismiss or disregard your wife's needs. You claim that you don't have to listen to her because you're the man. So, you do what you want. Looking at it this way, I suggest that both of you are in control. That's the good news. The bad news is that both of you are also out-of-control. Neither of you are getting what you want, and neither of you are giving in. In this sense you both share the same conflict about control: each of you needs control, but at the same time are sabotaging any chance of getting it; at least for the long-term. Both of you are working at cross purposes.

In this section I joined the couple by suggesting that they are both in and out-of-control. This maneuver helped them to see the futility of their positions and that their options are limited. I also tried to show them, with an old metaphor in mind: "The grass will not always be greener on the other side of the fence."

Step 3. Broadening the Context of the Conflict

To help Shanice and Deshawn better appreciate their shared conflict, I pointed out the role it plays in the broader context of their lives. One of the best places to begin this process is a person's place of employment. If a person does not like to be controlled, it will often show at work.

Therapist: Deshawn, how's it going at work?

Shanice: That's a great question. Tell him Deshawn.

Deshawn: You know . . . it's okay.

Shanice: Don't lie to the man . . . because I'll walk out right now.

Deshawn: The Principal and Superintendent get on me. They need everything done yesterday.

Shanice: Yeah, and Deshawn needs to do everything next year.

Therapist: So, you're having the same problem at work that you have at home?

Deshawn: I don't know.

Therapist: Anywhere else?

Shanice: If the kids need him to take them somewhere, Deshawn is always too busy. They can't count on him.

Therapist: How about you Shanice? My bet is that you are taking charge at work and probably overworking. Just an educated guess.

Shanice: This is a problem I've had forever. I just don't trust anyone else to do the job, so if I need one done and done right, I do it myself.

Therapist: So, when do you relax? If you cannot delegate responsibility, when do you take a break?

Shanice: (Tearful) Never . . . I've taken care of my mother and siblings. And now I've got even more responsibility and can't get help from my husband.

Therapist: Yeah, but even though they appreciate you, I'll also bet your bosses have encouraged you to delegate a little more.

Deshawn: They have . . . they call her the "general."

Some couples therapists are concerned about being too confrontative with a couple. Knowing when to intervene and how hard to challenge a couple's defensive structure is important. One confrontational technique I use is to invite the partner who I am not challenging to weigh in. I do not allow them to piggyback on my intervention to the point that the treatment becomes unbalanced, but I may carefully enlist them to help me break down their partner's defenses. Notice that I allowed Shanice to help me to get Deshawn to admit that he has the same trouble at work that he does at home. I did not do the same with Deshawn only because Shanice was more forthcoming, and I did not want the animosity between the two partners to escalate.

Step 4. Examining Each Partner's Family of Origin

Shanice grew up in a single parent household consisting of her mother and three younger siblings (two brothers and a sister). Shanice barely remembers her father and she has only seen him around town now and then. She also claimed that he never sent money and that she and her mother worked hard to support the family, sometimes holding down four or five jobs between the two. Shanice, as the oldest sibling, was parentified (Boszormenyi-Nagy & Spark, 1973) and learned to be responsible at an early age. She was also very smart and a great student. Shanice was offered a scholarship, completed her degree, and followed up with a master's degree in human resources.

Deshawn was also the product of a single-family household. He said that his parents were never married but that he does see his father now and then. Deshawn was the youngest child of three siblings. He had two older sisters who he described as his mother's lieutenants. Deshawn said he did not mind his mother acting like the boss so much, but he did not like being ordered around by his sisters. He said that he felt bullied at times to do more around the house. He thinks his sisters were jealous because his mother let him do as he pleased. The following exchange was an attempt to connect the couple's respective families of origin to their current control struggle and their associated problems with domestic chores. Both should be somewhat obvious by now, but they initially were not clear to Deshawn and Shanice.

Therapist: Sounds like you grew up in a matriarchal home where the women were in charge.

Deshawn: They thought they were.

Therapist: What's that mean?

Deshawn: I didn't pay a lot of attention to them.

Therapist: I thought you minded your mother.

Deshawn: Not really. What I meant was that I understood why she was trying to boss me around. I didn't say I liked it or listened to her.

Therapist: Sounds familiar.

Shanice: It sure does. They needed him like I do, but they couldn't get much out of him. I blame it on his mother. She let him off the hook.

Therapist: Did you avoid them as well Deshawn?

Deshawn: I was out a lot.

Therapist: You've been running from women your whole life. How about the mother of your first three children?

Shanice: She was always hitting on him for more child support, but she's gone now. I took her job over too. I'm raising them.

Therapist: While you are to be admired Shanice, it looks like you are locked into a pattern as well.

Shanice: You mean I'm overworking again.

Therapist: Yes, and I think you're trying to take control over everyone's job. And it looks like this is okay with you, Deshawn, especially if she asks little of you.

The influences from each partner's family of origin in this case were easy to figure out. Shanice, the oldest sibling, was enlisted by her mother as a caretaker and she has been carrying this burden ever since. Deshawn, the baby of his family and the only male, has been running from control since his childhood days. These backgrounds were made for a conflict about control.

Step 5. Integrating Internal Conflict and Increasing Differentiation

Shanice wants more control over her environment and needs Deshawn to help her get it. But from his perspective, Shanice wants to control him the way his mother and sisters tried as a child and young adult, and he is battling this effort in real time. It makes sense that Deshawn is making this an issue about masculinity. For example, although he seems to have little love for his abandoning father,

Deshawn still sees him as a masculine role model who does what he pleases. But it is even more complicated. Deshawn was controlled to a certain extent in his family of origin, but he was also taken good care of. This, in my opinion, produced a master conflict about control: While he wants to be taken care of, he does not want to be told what to do; while he wants to be babied, he wants to be treated like a man.

Shanice's parentification has helped to create in her a conflict about control: While she wants to be in charge, she does not want to be burdened; while she wants control, she does not want all the responsibility. The following is a short segment in which I help the couple to integrate their shared conflict about control to reduce their issues with domestic chores:

Therapist: Deshawn, you seem to hate it when a woman nags you. But I think you're a bit more complex than that. This is your second marriage, and it tells me that you like being married. The problem here is that you also run from certain responsibilities that come with the institution. I'm not siding with Shanice, but you can get married ten more times and you're going to run into the same problem. I know your mother and sisters rode you to be more responsible, but I also know you love them and give them credit for raising you. Can you give the same credit to your father?

DeShawn: Forget my dad.

Therapist: But do you see what I'm driving at?

DeShawn: Yeah, I can't commit halfway. I'm either in or out.

Therapist: You got it. Few women would take your deal, and many would react even worse. I'm not suggesting that you emasculate yourself. But I am suggesting that you will have to give up some control to your wife and help her out. At first it will feel as if you're back home with your mother and sisters, but ultimately, you'll have even more control over your life because your relationship with Shanice will stabilize. I can't see any other options. Shanice is overloaded and is not backing down. I doubt you enjoy having an angry wife at home.

Deshawn: So, you think I'm still running from my mother and sisters?

Therapist: In a way, yes.

Deshawn: (Shifting stance) Shanice is a great woman. But she needs to use a different tone with me and maybe I'll be more likely to help.

Shanice: Deshawn I have tried everything. I don't want to torture you.

Deshawn: Okay, I get it.

Therapist: Look Shanice, I think that when you play the mother role to Deshawn nothing good comes of it. It only serves to keep you parentified because he runs from you, and you then feel less in control of your life. I know that you're used to being in charge, but you're also feeling burned out. You have been working incredibly hard since you were a young girl. I get it. But I doubt you want to repeat those days.

Shanice: No way. As I've said, I don't want to pressure Deshawn or emasculate him. I just want a working relationship.

Therapist: Then you'll have to give up some control.

Shanice: What does that look like?

Deshawn: Don't take over everything, and when I do help try not to criticize me. Accept some of my ways of doing things.

Shanice: If that's what it will take, I'll lay back. But you better step up.

Deshawn: Do you see how she just talked to me? That's what I'm talking about.

Therapist: I heard it, Deshawn. This may be harder than you think, Shanice. Remember, you were the go-to person in your family of origin. To combat parentification in adulthood you would have to give up some of that special attention you received by being the only competent one.

Shanice: Oh, I'm ready.

Therapist: We'll see.

Deshawn and Shanice were alike in that both shared a conflict around control. Each wanted control over their lives but had no clue how to get it on a consistent basis. Shanice derived specialness from being a caretaker but was also in danger of burning out. Deshawn wanted to be "the man" but he was not fond of responsibility. To achieve internal integration around control, Shanice had to grieve the loss of her childhood, give up some of the power and specialness she had in her family of origin, allow herself to delegate responsibility, and to learn how to approach Deshawn in a less parental manner. For Deshawn to achieve this goal, he had to understand that the concept of true masculinity does not mean that he can do whatever he wants, especially in marriage. In this sense he will have to give up his definition of a man as he knew it. It was not a matter of "either or" for Shanice or Deshawn, but rather a commitment to better balance and integrate the two sides of each of them regarding control. The next case is the last in which a couple presents with a nonsexual symptom.

Ganesh and Indira: Nonsexual Symptom—Staying Married (See Figure 6.3)

Ganesh and his wife, Indira, are a Hindu couple in their mid-30s. They have been married for two years and are successful engineers who work at different companies. Although their marriage was arranged in India, they initially claimed to be happy with the match. Both partners said that they liked each other and were physically attracted at first sight.

The chief complaint was that Indira wanted to have children and Ganesh was not sure he wanted to stay married. His main reason was that Indira was, in his words "modernized," and that she was constantly fighting with his parents over Hindu traditions. Ganesh's parents were very traditional and put pressure on the

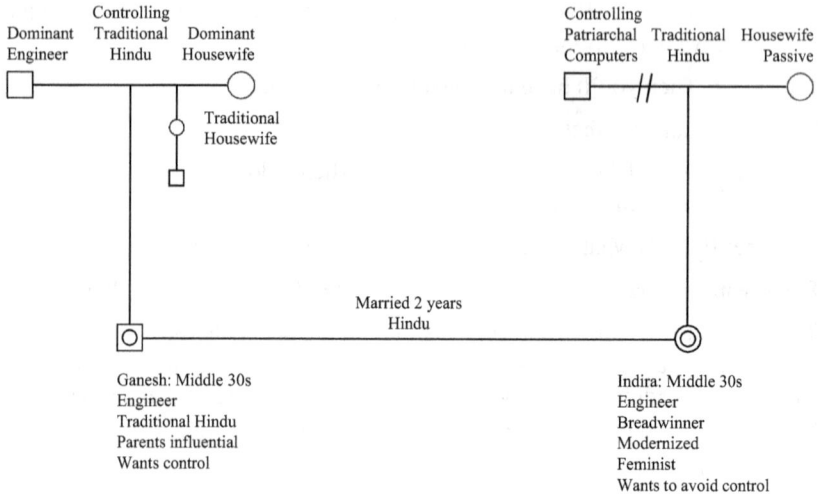

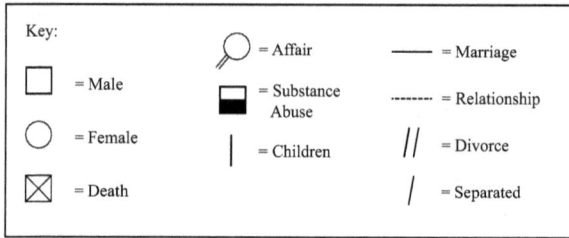

Figure 6.3   Ganesh and Indira.

couple to have children almost as soon as they married. They also did not appreciate that Indira voiced her opinion freely and often disagreed with their son.
They felt she was disrespectful and that she should play more of a subservient
role in her marriage.

Approximately 85% of the people in India still favor arranged marriages
and believe that a woman's place is in the home (Cultural India, 2017). Indira,
however, disagreed. She was a very bright woman who preferred the western-
ized culture of the United States. She enjoyed her freedom and the prestige she
earned as a professional. She relished a good intellectual debate and liked to
speak her mind. She earned more money than her husband and did not think that
she should be treated as his inferior.

Indira's interpretation of the couple's problem was that her husband had no
voice when it came to his parents. She was tired of his caving into them and
allowing them so much control over their lives. Ganesh claimed that he had
no trouble with his parents' values because he shared them. He wished that
Indira would give in and act more like a traditional Hindu woman. This control

struggle between Indira and Ganesh was the reason behind Ganesh's flirtation with divorce. He hated fighting with his parents.

According to Lee and Park (2013), the values inherent in therapy often come into conflict with the values of a multicultural population. The authors therefore recommend that the therapist should strive to become culturally competent. This would entail developing the "awareness, knowledge, and skills to intervene effectively in the lives of culturally diverse backgrounds" (p. 6). Lee (2013) called for the therapist to be open-minded and one who "simultaneously acknowledges human similarity and celebrates human differences" (p. 17). I try not to inflict my values onto a couple. Because each partner has two sides engaged in an internal battle, taking a side on almost any matter would only serve to exacerbate the couple's imbalance and increase their symptoms.

Step 1. Exposing the Couple's Control Struggle

I never thought that Ganesh wanted to leave Indira. My belief was that he found her too attractive, interesting, and smart. I suspected that he was hoping that by threatening to leave her he might exert enough pressure to back her down. But this tactic seemed to make Indira even more locked into her cause for gender equality. In the following dialogue I expose this and frame it as a control struggle:

Indira: Ganesh is ruled by his parents. He does not have a mind of his own. They are old fashioned and believe that men are superior to women. I make more money than Ganesh and I have more education (Ganesh has a bachelor's degree in engineering and Indira holds a master's in engineering). I do not think I should walk behind him when we go out and I will not raise a daughter to think that way. We no longer live in India.

Ganesh: When you remarry you can raise your daughter anyway you want.

Indira: That is all you have to say on the subject. You threaten me but you cannot negotiate.

Ganesh: My parents are in their 80s and you are upsetting them.

Therapist: Ganesh, what did you like about Indira when you married her?

Ganesh: I thought she was smart and beautiful.

Therapist: Do you still think of her that way?

Ganesh: Yes, I do.

Therapist: So, by your threats are you saying that it is worth divorcing your wife rather than disappointing your parents?

Ganesh: I worry about them.

Therapist: Hypothetically, suppose they come around to Indira's point of view. Since you say you share their values, would you still consider divorce?

Ganesh: Probably not.

Therapist: Why not? Unless you really do not want a divorce.

Ganesh: Well, sometimes I don't. But I must protect my parents.

Indira: That's interesting.

Therapist: So, your threats are for the most part, to get help from Indira with your parents.

Ganesh: That's what I really want, but she will not help. She makes things worse.

Therapist: Yes, but I see you both as vying for control. Ganesh, you need to get control over Indira for fear of upsetting your parents and causing a divorce. And you, Indira, you want Ganesh, but you are not willing to sacrifice your personal values to keep him.

Two important moments in this exchange came when Ganesh let it be known that he wanted Indira, but that he needed her help with his parents. To me this was an acknowledgement from him that his parents were difficult and served as a good segue into discussing the couple's conflict.

Step 2. Exposing the Couple's Conflict With Control

This conflict about control is obvious: Ganesh wants Indira to cooperate with his parents and follow a traditional Hindu lifestyle; he is trying for the sake of his parents to get her under control. Indira favors a feminist model; she is trying to avoid being controlled and in fact, wants her husband to adopt a freer model of living. But as is usually the case with control, the more each partner attempts to gain control, the less each has. In this case both partners are risking the loss of their marriage. The following is an example of how I exposed the couple's conflict to them:

Ganesh: If Indira would cooperate this would be over, and we could start a family. But I will not do so under these conditions. Any children we have will need their grandparents.

Indira: If you would stop putting your parents ahead of me this would all be over.

Ganesh: You are disrespectful to them. They are old and I love them.

Indira: They are disrespectful to me. Do you care at all about that?

Therapist: I know that both of you are under pressure to have a family. And your standoff is delaying this.

Ganesh: That is what I am saying.

Therapist: Yes, I know you want control of Indira, but this will not lead you to a family.

Indira: I want children very much, but Ganesh must put me first.

Therapist: Okay, so both of you would like to avoid divorce and to start a family. But instead of negotiating you are both wasting precious time and creating more animosity. In the end, nobody will have control—not even your parents, Ganesh.

This is a symmetrical couple with each partner clashing head-to-head and getting nowhere. I helped them to realize that they are both stubborn and that they needed to learn how to negotiate a compromise. Their manipulation of and complaining about one another is futile.

Step 3. Broadening the Context of the Conflict

Because the couple were locked into a specific context, I felt that broadening this would be especially valuable. The following is a brief example of how I showed the couple that their issue extends beyond their relationship:

Ganesh: Indira has a history of being rebellious. She fights with everybody.

Indira: I do not fight with everybody.

Therapist: Do you have a history of battle?

Indira: Because I fight for what I believe in, I have had many disagreements. My culture discriminates against women and so I have had to learn to fight for my rights.

Ganesh: That is only a part of it. You fight with friends and your own family. You have always been in one fight or another. It cannot be everybody else but you.

Therapist: Are you a revolutionary, Indira?

Indira: (Chuckling) I guess I am. But Ganesh has always been a controlling person. He is a rule follower, even if he does not believe in what he is supporting.

Therapist: Is that true, Ganesh? Do you follow the rules no matter how you truly feel about the situation?

Ganesh: I have been well schooled. I have been raised to study hard and to get good grades; to avoid trouble and to become a successful professional and to raise a family. These things are not all bad.

Therapist: You're right, but that wasn't the question. Do you do things that you do not agree with, just to appease someone?

Ganesh: I guess so. I do listen to my parents.

Therapist: Can you give me an example of when you listened to them against your better judgement?

Ganesh: The best example is that I wanted to come to the United States to study medicine—I really wanted to be a physician. But my father wanted me to be an engineer, like he was. He felt strongly that engineers were better at mathematics and science. He also believed that engineers create things that help society, unlike medicine where you treat one person at a time. My mother agreed.

This information was extremely valuable to the progress of the case. Indira did have a history of turmoil that transcended her conflicts with her husband and in-laws. And Ganesh had a history of following rules even if he disagreed with them. His story about medical school was especially sad and telling. Ganesh simply did not like to upset anybody, and this held true well beyond pleasing his parents. Let's see where these tendencies come from.

Step 4. Examining Each Partner's Family of Origin

Ganesh is the oldest of two siblings. He comes from an upper-caste traditional Hindu family where men rule. His father was a software engineer, and his mother was a housewife. Ganesh's parents put great pressure on him to do well in school and to marry and start a family with a Hindu woman. According to Indira, Ganesh grew up with many rules—first among them to please his parents.

Indira is an "only child." Her father was a computer analyst, and her mother was a housewife. Indira grew up in an unusual situation for a Hindu: her parents were divorced when she was young. She saw her mother experience a lot of discrimination being a single divorcee and considered that unfair. Indira promised herself that she would become a professional woman so that she did not have to depend on a man, and so she could feel free to express herself. Indira's father did stay involved in Indira's life, but he encouraged her to become a traditional Hindu wife. He and his ex-wife wanted Indira to marry a Hindu and have children. In the following segment I will demonstrate how I tied each partner's family of origin influences to their shared conflict about control in real time:

Therapist: Indira, it sounds as if your experience in your family of origin helped you to become the free and assertive woman you are. Your cultural experiences and your mother's plight proved influential.

Indira: Yes, absolutely.

Therapist: But aside from their divorce, your parents were quite traditional. And you did go along with them and your culture enough to agree to an arranged marriage. I suspect you're a little bit of each: revolutionary and traditionalist, or you never would have married Ganesh.

Indira: (Chuckles) That's probably true. I am a hybrid of sorts. Maybe I am a little confused because of my past.

Therapist: Maybe . . . and Ganesh, you were raised to be a traditional Hindu man in your family of origin. You respected your parent's control, but at times you also longed to make your own decisions. If you were able to make independent decisions, perhaps you would be a physician today. Not that being an engineer is a bad thing, but it wasn't your dream. Look, I know your marriage was arranged but you did know Indira, and you looked forward to marrying her. I also know that you could tolerate greater equality in your marriage if your parents sanctioned it.

Ganesh: I think I could, but we would have to find a way that will not devastate my parents.

Therapist: There is always some loss with compromise, but perhaps the three of us could work together to minimize this.

Because this couple were curious and highly intelligent, when they stopped battling long enough to open their ears, they learned something about themselves and their relationship. They especially saw just how much influence their upbringings have had on their current situation. I will expand this understanding even further in the next section.

Step 5. Integrating Internal Conflict and Increasing Differentiation

Ganesh was heavily influenced by his family to the point that he was in conflict about following their rules. For example, they were happy Indira was a Hindu, but they were a little concerned about the match. Ganesh liked Indira and was very attracted to her. He pushed the arrangement through, but he might have exaggerated what little traditional tendencies Indira possessed. Ganesh demonstrated an internal conflict: he wanted to control his own life choices, and he was intrigued by Indira's ability to rebel when she saw fit. But at bottom, he was a rule-follower.

Indira was rebellious and fought perceived injustice at every turn. But despite her somewhat unorthodox upbringing given her culture, her parents wielded some influence over her. Both her parents wanted her to marry a Hindu and to start a family as soon as possible. She was conflicted about having her independence and living a western lifestyle versus fulfilling a woman's traditional role in Hindu society. The integration process will be illustrated in the following example:

Therapist: I think you two are more alike than you think.

Indira: (Laughs) Really, I think we are as far apart as can be.

Therapist: Well, not really. I think you both want to please your parents and follow the rules to a certain extent. But Indira, you want to also be treated as an equal, especially by your husband. I suspect you liked Ganesh from the beginning because you got a sense that he could relate to your struggle. And Ganesh, you admittedly approved the match to Indira even though you knew something of her personality. That tells me that a part of you admired her ability to assert herself, even though it conflicted with your rule-following nature. You saw some of her traditional tendencies and perhaps you exaggerated them, but this is probably because you wanted her.

Indira: Okay, if we wanted each other and we are so alike, how come we are stuck with this conflict?

Therapist: Because you didn't know how alike you are on a conscious level. Instead of joining together to battle your shared conflict, you see each other on opposite sides of the fence and are unable to empathize.

Indira: So how do we get out of this?

Therapist: First each of you must acknowledge and take responsibility for your respective internal conflicts around control and realize that you cannot bully each other into submission. The thing you two are trying to conquer is the trait that has attracted you to each other. Why try to destroy it? It would be worth it to see if you both can integrate the two sides of this conflict and rebalance it in a way that is more functional. Then you can move on and start the family that you both want.

Fortunately, there was a strong enough bond between these two partners for them to go through the process of differentiation and invest in their marriage. Ganesh was not opposed to having an outspoken wife, but he needed to separate his desires from his parents' needs. He learned that he could not bully his wife into submitting to his parent's cultural expectations and that he needed to compromise with her instead. In doing so, he would probably suffer somewhat from his parent's reactions, but so be it. He would at least save his marriage and be able to start a family. I also suspect that he would not have to give in to Indira all the time. There was a part of Indira that was traditional and quite capable of allowing him to be in control in certain circumstances.

Indira needed to differentiate from her mother who she felt was treated unfairly, and to work with Ganesh rather than bully him into disregarding his parents completely. She specifically needed to be able to embrace some of her cultural traditions without fear of being dominated. To accomplish this, Indira would have to alter her revolutionary stances somewhat. Perhaps she can pick her battles and convey her points with a little less attitude.

Robert and Jonathan: Sexual Symptom— Male Hypoactive Sexual Desire Disorder (See Figure 6.4)

Robert and Jonathan are two gay men in their late 30s who have been together for 18 years and legally married for approximately three years. Jonathan is a professor of history at a local college and Robert is a chemical engineer. Jonathan insisted that Robert join him in treatment, or he threatened to bring another lover into their relationship. Robert apparently suffered from MHSDD. He claimed that he never had a great deal of sexual desire and that his problem is not specific to Jonathan. Robert rarely fantasizes but when he does, he claims to think about Jonathan, and to climax. He finds Jonathan physically attractive but he rarely, if

Nice
Successful   Over-   Conservative   Disengaged
Loose   achievers Religious   No structure
Boundaries Perfectionist Withholds   Workaholic   Chaos

Competitive
Close Knit

Married 3 years
Gay Couple

Robert: Late 30s   Jonathan: Late 30s
Chemical Engineer   Professor
Homophobic   Outgoing
Avoids being controlled   Handsome
Role model   Charismatic
Somewhat parentified   Angry
Perfectionist   Wants more control

Chief Complaint: Robert has MHSDD

Key:

◯ = Affair	─── = Marriage	
☐ = Male	▬ = Substance Abuse	----- = Relationship
◯ = Female	│ = Children	∥ = Divorce
⊠ = Death		╱ = Separated

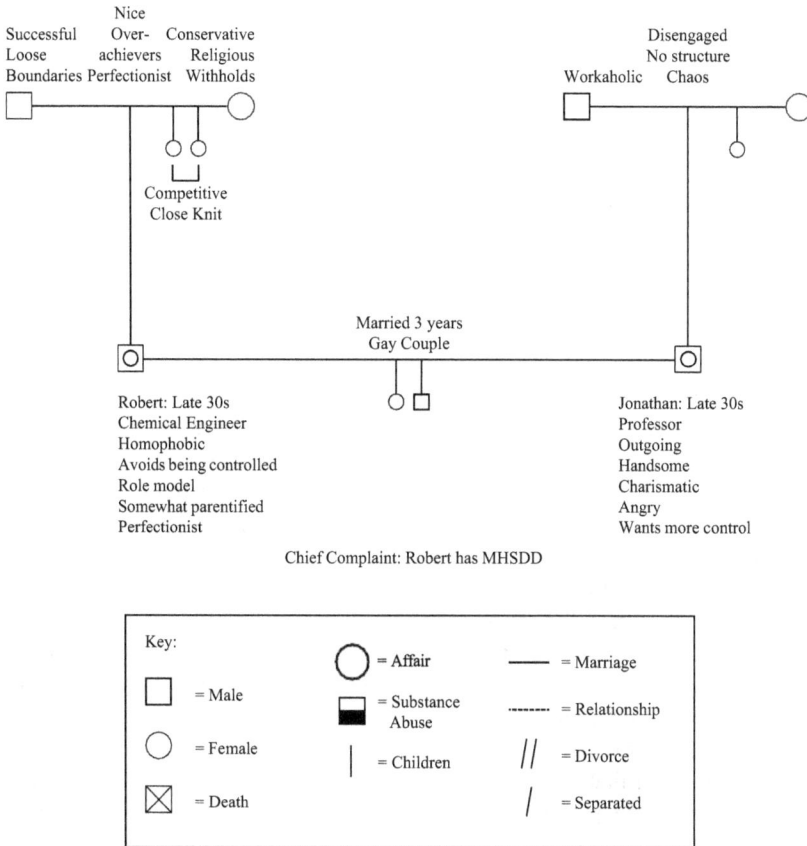

Figure 6.4   Robert and Jonathan.

ever, initiates sex. If Jonathan did not push Robert to discuss their sex life, Robert would admittedly let the issue die. Jonathan is getting tired of being the initiator and as a result, the couple's sexual frequency is even lower than it once was.

Robert and Jonathan get along in every other aspect of their life together. There is no history of sexual abuse or substance abuse or dependency. Robert did have some difficulty coming out, whereas Jonathan has been out for many years. In fact, Jonathan has an extensive history of gay relationships, and lived with another man for several years at a time. Although Robert did date and have sex with a couple of women during his college days, he claimed that he never really enjoyed it. He knew on some level that it was not right for him. Robert said that for the longest time he never considered being with a man, and that he disliked gays. He had to reconsider when, to his surprise, he developed a strong crush on a former boss. But even then, he would only allow for the possibility that he might be bisexual; he saw this as less stigmatizing. On the other hand, Jonathan was the sexual pursuer in the relationship (Betchen, 1997, 2005).

He relentlessly tried to get Robert to fully commit to being a gay man. Robert resisted avoiding what he perceived as Jonathan's pressure to trap him into a gay lifestyle. The chief way he did so was to develop a low libido.

The *Diagnostic and Statistical Manual of Mental Disorders* (5th ed.; *DSM-5*) (American Psychiatric Association, 2013) defines MHSDD as: (1) persistent deficient (or absent) sexual/erotic thoughts or fantasies and desire for sexual activity; (2) having symptoms persist for a minimum of six months; (3) causing significant distress; and (4) not better explained by a nonsexual mental disorder. It can be categorized as "lifelong" or always present; "acquired" or developed after a period of normal sexual functioning; "generalized" or not limited to certain situations or partners; and "situational" which only occurs with certain types of stimulation, situation, or partners (pp. 440–441).

The prevalence of MHSDD has been found to range from 15–25% (Lewis et al., 2010; Meana & Steiner, 2014). In a more recent study of approximately 4,955 men and women, Briken et al. (2020) reported that over one-third or 27.9% of the men surveyed experienced MHSDD during their lifetimes, with 14.7% experiencing the problem one year prior to the study. Approximately 12.0% of the men experienced the disorder from the beginning of sexual activity, and 64.5% experienced it in specific situations.

Older men are more prone to MDSDD disorder (Eplov et al., 2007; Fugl-Meyer et al., 1999). Briken and his colleagues reported that the disorder was found to be severely impairing as age increased: ages 18–25 = 10.4%; 46–55 = 14.3%; and 66–75 = 22.6%. And the rates of MHSDD in gay men (32.4 %) are similar those rates in heterosexual men (Peixoto & Nobre, 2016). Nimbi et al. (2020) concluded that the two groups did not differ on partner-related sexual desire within the couple, but factors such as negative stereotypes and stigmatization do influence how gay men express and interpret their desire.

According to Bhasin and Basson (2015), medical causes of MHSDD may include androgen deficiency, use of medications such as SSRIs, antiandrogens, gonadotropin-releasing hormone (GnRH), antihypertensives, anticonvulsants, and cancer chemotherapeutic agents. Psychological problems have been found to have an influence on MHSDD such as anxiety and depression (Clayton & Ramamurthy, 2008; Carvalheira et al., 2014), as well as various relationships issues including anger and resentment of one's partner (Corona et al., 2004), and intimacy issues (Weeks & Gambescia, 2015). Stress and trauma (Raisanen et al., 2018) as well as negative religious and cultural messages and sexual shame may also be factors (Hall & Graham, 2014; Woo et al., 2012).

Low sexual desire is one of the most difficult sexual disorders for couples therapists to contend with (Gambescia et al., 2021). Interventions that are routinely used include: anxiety and distress-reduction, providing psychoeducation, promoting communication, Sensate Focus exercises, improving sexual repertoire, simmering, and cognitive behavioral therapy (CBT) (Hall, 2020; Gambescia et al., 2021).

Using Robert and Jonathan as a case example I will illustrate how MHSDD can develop and be maintained in the context of a control struggle emanating from internal conflicts in each partner's family of origin. Consider the following 5-step process:

Step 1. Exposing the Couple's Control Struggle

This couple's control struggle was easy to detect. Jonathan pursued Robert for sex and Robert did what he could to avoid what he perceived as Jonathan's attempt to pressure and control him. The following exchange demonstrates how I exposed and framed the couple's control struggle:

Jonathan: Robert shows little interest in me, and I'm not used to that.

Therapist: Meaning?

Jonathan: I've never experienced this before. Most men are attracted to me. I've never had to chase anyone down to have sex.

Robert: You don't have to chase after me.

Jonathan: When was the last time you ever initiated sex?

Robert: I'm not as assertive as you.

Jonathan: (Rolling his eyes) Please.

Therapist: Robert, what do you think Jonathan should do?

Robert: I don't know. But he is constantly on my back about this.

Therapist: Are you admitting that nothing he can do will work?

Robert: I don't know.

Jonathan: He's in total control of our sex life. There's nothing I can do about it other than to leave him or take a lover. I've been thinking about my options.

Therapist: That's okay Robert, you don't have to know what's going on right now, but it sounds as if you're at least admitting that you can't give Jonathan what he needs sexually.

Robert: I guess so. But I don't feel in control because he is torturing me.

Jonathan: I'm torturing you because you control our sex life or lack thereof, and it's not fair.

This is not an unusual exchange for a couple in which one partner has low sexual desire. In my experience, the symptom-bearer is fighting off feeling sexually controlled but does not see himself in control at all. In fact, most seem to have no idea where their desire has gone or what to do about it. Typically, the other partner, if male, feels emasculated, and uses every technique to get the symptom-bearer to show interest. This partner needs more control over their sex life. But the more he pursues, the more resistant or distanced the symptom-bearer becomes. In this case, Robert wants Jonathan to leave him alone and allow him to exist in a sexless relationship, and Jonathan will not comply; he wants Robert to take more sexual responsibility. This is a dynamic that will end in neither party having a sufficient control. And if Jonathan follows through with taking a lover against Robert's wishes, the chaos will only escalate. In the next step I will expose the couple's conflict with control:

Step 2. Exposing the Couple's Conflict With Control

Therapist: Jonathan, it seems to me that you're trying to gain some control over your sex life, and Robert, you're trying to avoid being controlled by Jonathan. But what's fascinating about the struggle for control is that in my experience, the more you struggle with it the less you will end up with.

Jonathan: What do you mean?

Therapist: I mean the way you have been doing things is not working and you are a smart guy. Why do you keep using the same tactic or approach time and again if it continues to fail?

Jonathan: I don't know what else to do.

Therapist: Well, you say you want control, but you chose a man who withholds sex from himself and from you. And then you pursue him, which only chases him away. These indicators tell me that you may have a conflict about getting the control that you want. And Robert, you control sex to the point that you risk Jonathan having an affair or leaving you. I would say that neither of you will end up with control in the end.

Jonathan: It feels that way. But why would we sabotage ourselves?

Therapist: That's a key question. But first let's explore your conflicts a bit more.

Step 3. Broadening the Context of the Conflict

Notice in the following exchange, how each partner expands the context of their problem. Jonathan speaks to Robert's difficulty getting close to anyone and how he controls even what limited friendships he has. Robert talks about Jonathan's neediness of people. Each partner is on the attack primarily to defend themselves, yet they are right about one another.

Therapist: Jonathan, I remember you said that you're not used to men who aren't attracted to you. Can you say more about that?

Jonathan: Not to sound narcissistic, but I've never had any trouble attracting men. But Robert won't even hold my hand or put his arm around me.

Therapist: So, he isn't very affectionate.

Robert: I'm like that with everybody.

Therapist: Do you both have friends?

Jonathan: All the friends we have are mine. Robert isn't that close to anybody.

Robert: I have friends, but they don't live close, so I rarely talk to them.

Jonathan: When was the last time you spoke to one of your friends?

Robert: I don't know.

Jonathan: Right.

Robert: Well, who has time for friends when Jonathan has people in and out constantly. Sometimes it's very annoying. He seems to need people around him all the time. He cooks for them as if he's holding court.

Therapist: The world beyond your sexual issue sounds similar. Robert, you seem to feel more in control when you have a certain amount of distance, and Jonathan you prefer when people are around.

Robert: It's the same way at work. Jonathan needs to work with people, and I can spend hours alone doing my job. I'd rather not be bothered.

Jonathan: Yeah, but Robert gets pressured sometimes by his boss to socialize with others at work, and he resists.

Robert: And you have your colleagues over the house every weekend, as if you don't see them enough during the work week. It's like you're anxious being alone.

Step 4. Examining Each Partner's Family of Origin

Robert was raised in a family in which he was the oldest of three siblings. His parents were described as nice people who pushed their children to succeed, and they all have. Although the siblings are scattered across the country they stay in contact via telephone and Internet.

Robert described his childhood as relatively uneventful aside from some intense sibling competition, but he said he usually handled that well. His parents often looked at him to be the role model for his siblings, and as a likeable individual and excellent student, he gladly excepted the role of the perfect young man.

Robert had little complaints about his family of origin and said that while they were open-minded, especially about topics such as sex. It was only later in the treatment that it finally came out that his father often complained about the lack of sex and his mother complained about her husband constantly wanting it. In fact, Jonathan added that Robert's father was horny enough to constantly make sexual jokes to their maid. Robert admitted he too, felt somewhat embarrassed by his father's behavior but that he knew he could do little about it. Now he is in a similar struggle.

Robert dated straight women here and there but had little sexual experience. He said that he was not turned on and that he preferred to only have sex with someone that he loved. He first considered that he was different during puberty but would only entertain the possibility that he could be bisexual. As mentioned, once he graduated college and took his first job, he found himself wildly attracted to his boss—a handsome straight man. This bothered Robert but he continued to reject the possibility that he was gay until he met Jonathan. Robert was more concerned with coming out than his family was. In fact, they were supportive of him and accepted Jonathan into the family immediately.

Jonathan was the oldest of two siblings. He claimed that he came out early. His childhood was far less structured, and he learned to please himself at an early age. His parents were accepting of his sexual orientation, but they were somewhat disengaged from his life. His father was a workaholic and his mother catered to his younger sister. Jonathan soon learned that he was considered very handsome and attractive to both men and women. Although he had a few brief relationships with women, most of his sexual experiences were with men.

People of all orientations found Jonathan likeable and charismatic. He loved having them around and having them close. When he first met Robert, he saw him as an attractive, bright man, but also as a "rookie" in the gay world who needed help with his homophobia, as Jonathan put it. He saw himself as Robert's tutor, but he ended up having less control over his star pupil than he anticipated. Next, we will see how the couple did when it came to integrating their conflict around control and increased their differentiation from their respective families of origin.

Step 5. Integrating Internal Conflict and Increasing Differentiation

Therapist: Robert, it sounds as if your father was a bit feisty.

Robert: (Giggles) You could say that.

Jonathan: He was downright horny.

Therapist: So, did his off-color jokes to the maid bother you?

Robert: He made me blush a few times.

Therapist: How did it make your mother feel?

Robert: She hated it. She would try and stop him, but he would just tell her that she was too uptight.

Therapist: So, would you say that at times, he was out-of-control?

Robert: You could say that.

Therapist: Does Jonathan make sexual jokes around you?

Robert: All the time. But he never embarrasses me in public. That's the difference.

Therapist: Yes, that's a significant difference but the dynamic is similar, isn't it?

Robert: I guess so.

Therapist: Can he be embarrassing at all . . . in a sexual sense?

Robert: Yes. He likes to explore and to be affectionate in public and that bothers me. I can't do that. I get too embarrassed.

Therapist: So, Jonathan wants more than you can give him.

Robert: Yes.

Therapist: Jonathan, it sounds like you're playing the role of Robert's father.

Robert: The truth is that Jonathan is a wild man. He will try or risk anything. He always ups-the- ante and it frightens me.

Therapist: He too, is a product of his upbringing? He can appear out-of-control?

Robert: Yes. Absolutely.

Therapist: So, your control struggle is about sexual boundaries. Robert, you want stricter sexual boundaries and Jonathan you want looser ones.

Robert: Yes, that's about right.

Therapist: Okay, but why would you choose each other? Robert, why not find someone with your sexual values? Why pick a man like Jonathan?

Jonathan: I can answer that. He was attracted to my charisma. He and his family are so provincial and sometimes downright boring.

Robert: And he needs family structure. He'd probably have an assortment of sexual diseases without me, and probably be financially broke.

Jonathan: (Laughs) Probably true.

Therapist: So, you both need something that simultaneously bothers each of you? Jonathan, you need structure and people around—you need a family, and Robert provides this. But because his perfectionistic family is so close, he cannot shake his need to be perfect. This feeds his homophobia and prevents him from his true self. And you, Robert, need Jonathan's free spirit, but it scares the hell out of you.

Jonathan: (Laughs) That's sick.

Therapist: It's called a conflict.

Jonathan and Robert were two very smart men, interested in saving their relationship. Despite his threats to end their relationship or to take a lover, Jonathan desperately needed a family and Robert came with one. Robert needed to accept himself and to be more spontaneous like his free-spirited mate. Jonathan had few rules and on an unconscious level this appealed to Robert who came from more of a controlled background. Only his father provided some chaos now and then. But Robert's distancing caused Jonathan pain; he has already experienced far too much distance in his life. And Jonathan's pressure was too much for Robert. He grew up with pressure.

Most of Jonathan's threats were posturing. Once he made the decision to allow himself to be vulnerable—without the defenses he used to protect himself from being abandoned—he was better able to differentiate enough to accept Robert's limitations. It was scary to him, but he eventually curbed his need to pressure Robert. Robert better differentiated from his perfectionism and allowed himself to be less self-critical. To accomplish this feat, he had to abandon or differentiate from the "perfect child" persona he inherited from his family of origin. In turn, this curbed his homophobia and allowed him to be more of the kind of sexual partner Jonathan wanted. Neither partner was completely satisfied, but each had enough control to move on and enjoy their life together.

MHSDD is a common sexual disorder, but delayed ejaculation is not. We will see how Sandy and Joel dealt with this complex issue in the context of control.

Sandy and Joel: Sexual Symptom—Delayed Ejaculation (See Figure 6.5)

Joel is a 55-year-old physician; his 45-year-old fiancée Sandy, is a freelance writer. The couple have no children even though they were both previously married; Joel is a divorcee and Sandy is a widow. While the couple live together and have been engaged for two years, they decided not to marry until they resolve Joel's delayed ejaculation. Joel can ejaculate by other means (with oral or manual stimulation) but never during intercourse with Sandy. This is the first time he has ever experienced this issue.

Although Sandy can achieve orgasm with clitoral stimulation, she is still quite upset about the situation. She believes Joel's symptom is a sign that he is not attracted to her. Oddly, Joel did not appear distraught at all. He decided to attend sessions primarily because he does not like that Sandy will not let the issue rest. Apparently, Sandy intermittently loses her temper and threatens to end the relationship.

Joel claims that he is physically attracted to Sandy. On the surface, this does not look as if the couple are engaged in a control struggle, but upon further examination, a sizeable one is revealed. In this control dynamic, Sandy uses emotional manipulation and verbal threats to secure a feeling of being in control; Joel is dismissive of his wife.

According to the American Urological Association (2020), delayed ejaculation is reserved for those men who experience trouble achieving climax during sexual activity. If the disorder has always been present it is referred to as "lifelong;" if there was a time that the client did not have the disorder, such as in Joel's case, it is said to be "acquired." The *DSM-5* (American Psychiatric Association, 2013) defines delayed ejaculation as: (1) a significant delay in ejaculation, and (2) a pronounced infrequency or absence of ejaculation lasting six months or more and occurring 75–100% of the time a couple participate in sexual activity. The reference has also categorized the disorder as "generalized:" meaning the client experiences the problem with every partner; or "specific:" meaning the partner experiences it only with their partner or specific person (pp. 424).

Delayed ejaculation is the least understood male sexual disorder (Perelman, 2020) with prevalence estimates for the general type at approximately 2.5% (Rowland & Kolba, 2018). Some common causes of the disorder are: aging (Abdel-Hamid & Ali, 2018), trauma (Rogers, 2019), intimacy, fear of pregnancy, negative messages about sex, relationship issues, ambivalence about sex, and hidden sexual preferences (Perelman & Watter, 2016). Certain medications

Anxious
Controlling
Critical   Confusing

Helpful
Kind

Incompetent
Hardworking
Distant

Babied Joel

She left

Engaged 2 years

Joel: 55 years old
Physician
Controlling
Babied

Sandy: 45 years old
Writer
Fun loving
Raised self
Little structure
Latchkey child

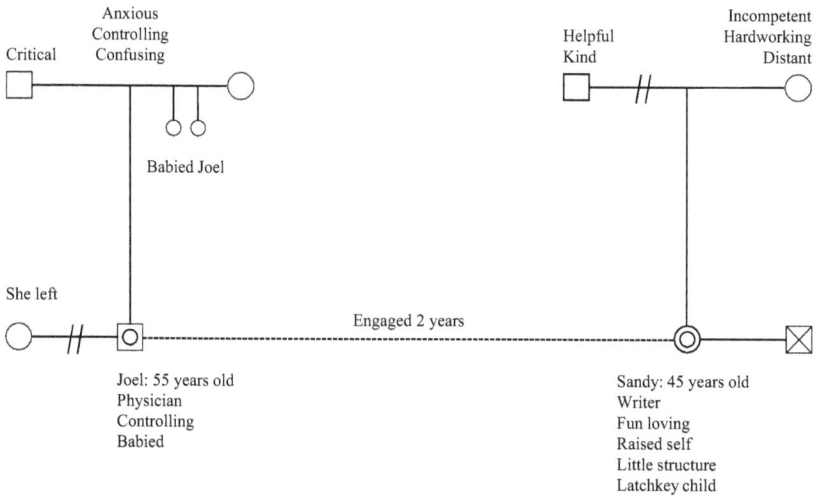

Chief Complaint: Joel's Delayed Ejaculation

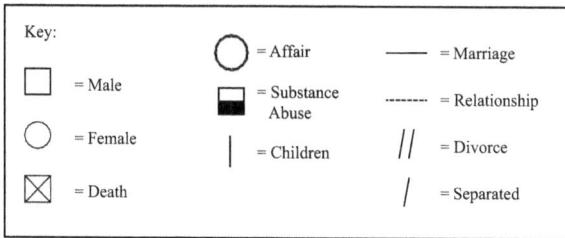

Key:

☐ = Male

◯ = Female

⊠ = Death

◯ = Affair

▧ = Substance Abuse

| = Children

——— = Marriage

------- = Relationship

// = Divorce

/ = Separated

Figure 6.5 Sandy and Joel.

may also be factors such as antiadrenergics, antihypertensives, and antipsychotics (Di Sante et al., 2016).

For many clinicians, the treatment of choice for delayed ejaculation is either cognitive behavioral therapy (Metz & McCarthy, 2007) or integrative therapy (Foley & Gambescia, 2020; Perelman, 2018). Betchen and Davidson (2018) demonstrated how to treat delayed ejaculation using MCT. The latter approach is used here to treat the disorder but with an eye on an underlying conflict with control. In the following vignette I expose the couple's control struggle:

Step 1. Exposing the Couple's Control Struggle

Therapist: So, Sandy, you're threatening to leave Joel over this problem.

Sandy: I don't want to, but he has been putting this off for a couple of years and I can't take it anymore.

Therapist: I understand your frustration.

Joel: I don't. She can have sex if she wants, and it's my orgasm that's affected, not hers.

Sandy: That's his excuse. He doesn't seem to realize how this affects me.

Therapist: Well, explain it to me again.

Sandy: I feel like he is lying about his attraction to me. I think he is more attracted to someone else. He ejaculates to porn. Why not with me?

Joel: That's not true. I can ejaculate with oral and manual sex with you.

Sandy: It's not the same. That feels robotic. Intercourse feels more intimate.

Joel: Maybe if you stopped threatening to leave, I could fix this.

Sandy: I've tried that, but you still do nothing.

Therapist: Why did you procrastinate in seeking treatment, Joel?

Joel: I was too embarrassed.

Therapist: That's a common reaction. But did it occur to you that you might be making things worse by ignoring it?

Joel: Sandy would still be angry. She is taking this very personally.

Sandy: That's because you won't even talk to me about it.

Therapist: So, it sounds like a standoff: Joel, you want Sandy to drop the subject. And Sandy, you have become increasingly tense and threatening. Neither of you can empathize. It seems to me that, as a couple, you are gridlocked.

If Joel would have at least voluntarily dealt with his delayed ejaculation he would not have exacerbated Sandy's anxiety and ire. But she is right; without her prodding he may never have entered treatment. And while Sandy may feel justified in her feelings towards Joel, rather than show empathy she has threatened to leave him time and again. Whether she wants to or not, the threat of abandonment is raising his anxiety and contributing to his dim view of her ability to empathize. Joel seems to want her to accept him unconditionally, but he makes it difficult for her to do so.

Step 2. Exposing the Couple's Conflict With Control

I believed Sandy when she said that she didn't want to leave Joel, but not for the reasons she cited. I saw her in conflict: A part of her was devastated that Joel could not ejaculate during intercourse, but rather than help the situation, she made it worse. To me this was a sign that she was ambivalent about a cure. Joel was holding back, but I also believed that he loved Sandy and wanted to settle down with her. I suspected that it would be easier to convince Joel of his conflict because Sandy saw herself as the clear-cut victim in this case. Let us see:

Therapist: I think you are in conflict, Joel. Do you know what I mean?

Joel: Not really.

Therapist: You seem to want to stay with Sandy, but you can't give all of yourself to her.

Joel: Yeah. I want to be with Sandy, but she makes it hard.

Therapist: Yes, quite a dilemma. And Sandy I see that you want Joel but his problem and the way he handles it is intolerable.

Sandy: I just want a normal life. If he at least worked on it, it would be easier deal with.

Therapist: I understand, but suppose his embarrassment is real?

It is not necessary to pathologize either partner to make a point about their control struggle. I simply present the struggle to them as if it is a problem for the couple system. This technique helps to join them rather than exacerbate their perceived difference.

Step 3. Broadening the Context of the Conflict

When sexual symptoms are present, it is much easier to distinguish between content and process because the symptom itself is the content. In this case, the symptom is delayed ejaculation. The downside to this, however, is that couples often become so focused on such a pronounced symptom they may resent and resist spending time on anything else. This is especially true now that most couples read about their symptoms on the Internet and determine on their own how they should be treated.

A competent colleague referred a couple to me after he was unceremoniously fired by them. In the first session, the couple confessed that they ended their treatment because my colleague insisted that if their relationship dynamics were adjusted their sexual symptom would most likely dissipate. He was probably right, but the couple thought he was wasting their time and money, and so they terminated him. Notice in the following vignette how I tied Joel and Sandy's sexual problem (content) to their nonsexual control struggle (process) in a way that neither feel that I am ignoring their wishes. Also note how much easier it was to then broaden their content.

Therapist: Sandy, you mentioned that Joel rarely compliments you.

Sandy: Actually, he's extremely critical of me. I know he's a perfectionist, but I'm not a loser.

Therapist: Can you give me an example of one of his criticisms?

Sandy: When I try to take something on, he rips me. For example, if I plan a vacation for us, he might tell me that I picked an awful place, and that I don't know how to choose a hotel. Then he takes over and claims to have fixed everything.

Therapist: He takes control?

Sandy: Yes, he does.

Therapist: So, Joel, you control more than just your ejaculate?

The therapist must take turns moving from process to content and back again throughout the therapeutic process. This will make it easier to show the couple that their issue is not limited to the specific symptom they are presenting. While this may be somewhat shocking to some couples, they will be relieved to know that they have only one constant problem rather than several problems.

Step 4. Examining Each Partner's Family of Origin

Joel was the oldest son of three siblings; he has two younger sisters. He said that his parents treated him special because he was the only son in a traditional Jewish family where boys are usually considered more valuable. He described his parents as very anxious and controlling individuals. He said that he was babied until he left for college. He also saw them as "confusing." He said that his father meant well, but that he would challenge all Joel's decisions. Sometimes his father called him "stupid" if he thought he made a bad decision or one that he did not approve of. Joel said that he was never angry with his father, but instead thought it was somewhat funny. He chuckled and admitted that he could be an idiot. Overall, he said that he gets along with his parents but now that he is older, he cannot take their criticisms on a regular basis. Ironically, Joel's first wife left him because she felt that he was too critical of her; she saw him as charming but somewhat abusive.

Sandy seconded the motion that Joel's parents are critical. She said that every time they visit, his father criticizes the structure of their home and his mother checks for dust. Sandy feels she will never be good enough for their "baby," and although she wants children, she dreads what they will say about her childrearing skills.

Sandy comes from a single-parent family. Her parents were divorced when she was a pre-teen, but she has maintained contact with her father who she claimed is exceedingly kind and helpful to her. Sandy said that because her mother held two jobs to make ends meet, she was a latchkey child. Unlike Joel, she was taught to live with less and to be tolerant of others. Sandy was also taught to be self-reliant, but there were few rules. She claimed that she basically raised herself and there was little control over anything. She said that she was even allowed to marry her first husband at 18-years-old. However, he died young of a heart attack and left her with little money.

Step 5. Integrating Internal Conflict and Increasing Differentiation

Joel came from a family of critical controllers. Nothing he did was ever good enough because they could do it better. But they did take good care of him. In fact, they infantilized him. While Joel did enjoy certain aspects of being treated special, he did not appreciate being controlled. He said that he could not wait to escape and go to college. After college he married, but his wife left him after a few years primarily because, as I have said, he was too critical and demanding. While Joel is somewhat less critical with Sandy, he still acts as if he always has a better idea; he is also demanding.

Sandy saw Joel as controlling of her, their money, and how much he commits to the relationship. His delayed ejaculation is symbolic of his withholding positive reinforcement, and it is a way that he maintains control over the relationship. It is not that Joel is not stimulated enough by Sandy—she is extremely attractive, as was his ex-wife. He also seems to enjoy having sex with her and their frequency is consistent. Because Joel was spoiled, he needs a woman to take care of him—a woman like Sandy—but he cannot allow her to control him. He was stuck in quite a conflict.

Sandy has had some bad luck in her life but has survived it all. Her parents divorced when she was young, and her late husband died unexpectedly. She has worked hard to survive and deserves credit, but Joel withholds positive reinforcement and is critical of her. Complicating matters, Sandy came from a broken family with few boundaries and little to no rules. She had to depend on herself. But while this was a hard life, it came with a lot of freedom. As a result, she does not appreciate being constantly criticized and told what to do. She does, however, need a family and a sense of security and Joel provides these for her. Sandy believes that her inability to bring Joel to orgasm is a sign that she will never get what she wants from him. She needs a family but not the control that sometimes comes with it. Notice how the couple responds when their control conflict is connected to their delayed ejaculation.

Therapist: Joel, it must be hard to fully commit to someone after your divorce?

Joel: I guess.

Therapist: Weren't you devastated?

Joel: Yes, I certainly didn't want to lose my wife.

Therapist: She did a lot for you didn't she?

Joel: Yes, she helped me through school and was my cheerleader. She treated me like a prince.

Therapist: Until she exiled you.

Joel: (Nervous chuckle) If it weren't so tragic it would be funny.

Therapist: You're used to being taken care of, but not without criticism. It seems to me that you traded your independence for a royal title of prince.

Joel: (Laughs) I can see that.

Therapist: Now that you have your freedom, you want a woman to treat you like a prince, but you cannot treat her like a princess. Instead, you seem to expect too much of her, and you belittle her the way your parents did you. Perhaps this is your way of never again giving anyone control over you. In doing so, however, you maintain your freedom but possibly lose another woman. Does this sound like a good deal to you?

Joel: No, I don't want to lose Sandy.

Therapist: Sandy, you have lost a lot in your life, and I cannot think of anyone who deserves a stable, loving relationship more than you do. You are not used to being criticized or controlled and you claim to despise both, yet you chose someone who has a history of controlling, critical behavior. Perhaps you have traded your freedom for the prospects of security and a stable family. You have even found a way to personalize the delayed ejaculation.

To balance his internal conflict Joel would have to give up being the prince he was raised to be—this would help to cut down on his criticisms and demands of Sandy. He would also have to get over his fear of losing control again to a woman and commit to Sandy, which in turn would help him to stop withholding from her. To do so, Joel would have to integrate being both in and out-of-control. He would not seem to have as much control as he would like on the surface, but by giving up some to Sandy he would have more in the end. Sandy would have to curb her desperate need to have a family and to value herself more. She could then refrain from personalizing Joel's criticisms as well as his delayed ejaculation. This in turn would allow her to feel more in control over her relationship and her life in general.

Sam and Marge: Sexual Symptom—Female Orgasmic Disorder (See Figure 6.6)

Sam and Marge are two divorcees in their late 50s that have dated many years and finally got the courage to marry. Sam was a civil engineer and Marge, an insurance underwriter. The couple decided to seek couples therapy because Marge could not achieve orgasm. She could reach climax with a vibrator, but never in the presence of a man or during intercourse.

While Marge admitted that she enjoyed foreplay and intercourse, at times she felt like giving up and never having sex again because of her inability to orgasm. She explained to Sam that it was nothing personal, but Sam was nevertheless distraught by Marge's sexual limitations. He said that he loved her and would never leave her, but he was unhappy with their sex life. Marge said that Sam's unhappiness often showed in his irritability and short temper with her. Sam claimed that Marge would retaliate by avoiding sex when she could, and by picking on him about anything she could find.

This couple demonstrated a symmetrical dynamic in that each openly fought for control. They both used the same techniques which were outlined

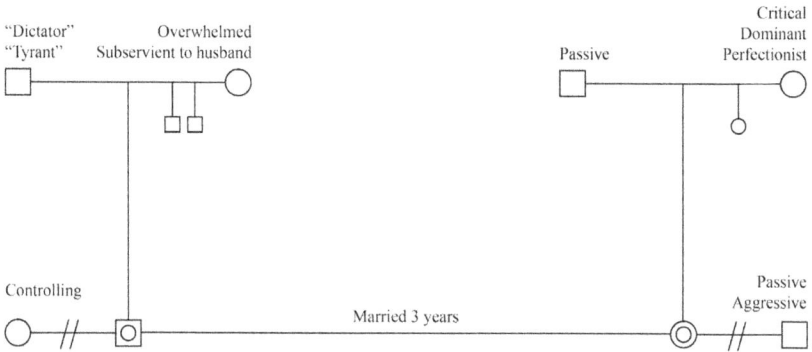

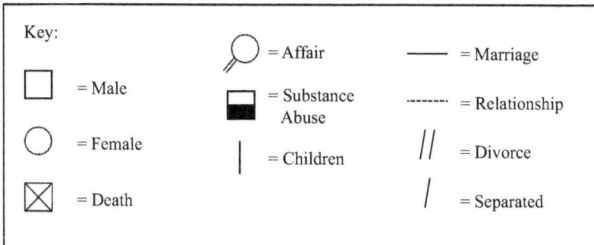

Figure 6.6   Sam and Marge.

in "Chapter 4. Controlling Styles" to gain control and avoid being controlled. Although insight was key in treating this case, it also merited the integration of sex therapy exercises. In the MCT model, exercises are usually not prescribed until the control struggle and internal conflict are exposed, and until the couple are comfortable enough in treatment to use them successfully; this usually takes place somewhere in *Step 5. Integrating Internal Conflict and Increasing Differentiation.*

The *DSM-5* (American Psychiatric Association, 2013) defines female orgasmic disorder as (1) a delay, infrequency, or absence of orgasm, and (2) a significant reduction of the intensity of orgasm. These symptoms must appear 75–100% of the time during sexual activity and persist for at least six months. As with other sexual dysfunctions, female orgasmic disorder can be lifelong or acquired as well as generalized or situational (pp. 429–430). Prevalence rates suggest that

45% of women reported achieving orgasm half of the time; one quarter reporting that they cannot reach orgasm 75% of the time; and 30% claiming that they can never achieve orgasm (Rowland & Kolba, 2016).

Briken et al. (2020) found that the rates of women with orgasmic problems were greater than that of delayed ejaculation in men: men ages 18–25 = 9.3% compared to women at 27.0%; men ages 36–45 = 8.8% compared to women at 28.4%. But as they aged, men reported higher rates of delayed ejaculation: ages 66–75 = 15.7% compared to women with orgasm problems at 11.6%. Let us now see how Sam and Marge navigated the 5-step treatment process.

Step 1. Exposing the Couple's Control Struggle

Although dedicated to each other, Sam and Marge were gridlocked in a control struggle beyond any others that I have seen in treatment, and they admitted it. But they never once mentioned the word "control."

Marge: Sam is so difficult to live with. He's constantly annoyed. He gets very frustrated with me because I can't orgasm.

Sam: I'm probably more upset that you avoid me.

Marge: I only avoid you because of your reaction. I can't take it anymore. Why don't you find someone who is perfect in bed?

Sam: You're not easy to live with either. You seem on edge all the time and you harass me to keep our place spotless. You've known from the beginning that I don't care about having a place that looks like it should be shown in a magazine.

Therapist: When is the last time you two have had sex?

Sam: Last month

Marge: Three weeks ago.

Therapist: And exactly what happened? Give me a video picture.

Sam: The usual: Marge controlled the process. She can only have sex in one position: missionary style. There's some oral foreplay from her, but I'm not allowed to pleasure her.

Marge: That's because it doesn't feel pleasurable. Do I have to do everything you see in the movies and magazines?

Sam: Anyway, we began intercourse and although Marge seemed initially into it, at some point she just shut down. I orgasmed and we fell asleep.

Marge: That wasn't all of it. You got aggressive sexually and tried to force me to orgasm.

Sam: Right, then you picked on me for the rest of the night.

Marge: You deserved it.

Therapist: So, this is the dance that the two of you have been gridlocked in for several years?

Marge: Yup.

Therapist: For some reason, Marge—which we haven't figured out yet—you are withholding your orgasm. And you, Sam, are trying to force an orgasm out of Marge. This looks like a long-standing control struggle that we must get to the bottom of.

Sam and Marge were both divorcees, and I could tell that neither were interested in parting. Marge was open to considering her control issues. Sam presented as a gruff, conservative man somewhat skeptical to psychotherapy. But I will say that he was game enough to give it a try and he did not seem like a quitter. He also seemed to be quite in love with Marge.

Step 2. Exposing the Couple's Conflict With Control

It soon became obvious that Marge did not like to give up control to anyone. She admitted that she was self-protective and hated being told what to do. But she also seemed to like strong, relatively accomplished men who were outspoken. Ironically, these men also made her feel out-of-control. Sam was a contrarian who insisted on doing things his way. This cost him his first marriage, and at times interfered with his career aspirations. But he also liked to battle strong, intelligent, opinionated women who ironically, were a threat his need for control.

Therapist: You two battle quite a bit.

Marge: Sam is always ready for a fight, and with our sex life the way it is, he is intolerable.

Sam: I want a good sex life. Is that too much to ask?

Marge: But you're angry and aggressive about it.

Sam: That's because you're controlling it.

Marge: I would love to have an orgasm.

Sam: But you argue and resist all the time.

Therapist: Sam, do you really think that your aggressiveness is helping your cause? From where I sit, your behavior doesn't gain you any control over your sex life. You're just in a perpetual wrestling match.

Sam: Yes, but she is tough.

Therapist: I agree that she is tough. You like tough women, but you can't stand being controlled. Do you see a conflict there? And you say you want sex but only seem to be aggravating Marge. Is this a new way of seducing a woman I should know about?

Sam: (Chuckles Nervously).

Therapist: Marge, you like strong men, but you wrestle them for control.

Marge: I know, it's a curse.

Marge and Sam are not just tough with each other—they're tough in treatment and attempt to battle with me over interventions. Nevertheless, perseverance and tolerance are key in exposing a couple's shared conflict. And with this couple, broadening their context is paramount to helping release them from gridlock.

Step 3. Broadening the Context of the Conflict

Broadening Sam's context was easier because he was also in control struggles with his friends, his career, and even his condominium association for failing to pay dues. Marge primarily did battle with her friends, and family.

Therapist: Do you like your profession Sam?

Sam: It's not bad. But dealing with some of the rules of the firm drive me crazy.

Marge: Oh, this will be fun. He's been called into his bosses' office so many times for ignoring their orders you'd think he doesn't care about keeping his job.

Therapist: I hear you also argue with friends.

Sam: Yeah well . . .

Therapist: And the condo association?

Marge: He owes them money. He just doesn't like to pay them.

Sam: It's a rip off.

Therapist: Okay, but conflict seems to make your world go around. Marge, do you have any friends?

Sam: Very few.

Therapist: And what about your sister?

Sam: She fights with all of them.

Marge: What can I say? I do not suffer fools gladly.

Step 4. Examining Each Partner's Family of Origin

Sam was the oldest of three brothers. His father was described as a "tyrant" who dictated Sam's every move, especially his career. His mother was overwhelmed with three boys and rarely challenged her husband. She too was under his control. Sam's first marriage produced no children, primarily because his ex-wife did not want any. Sam was upset by this but instead of leaving her he admittedly stayed on and tortured her over it. Sam described his first marriage as a battlefield and that his ex-wife was controlling enough to make Marge look submissive. He said when he and his first wife decided to divorce, his lawyer told him that his was the longest, nastiest, most expensive divorce he had ever witnessed.

Sam had an uneventful sex life. He dated frequently, engaged in a couple of long-term relationships, and married his first wife soon after he completed college. He divorced after 25 years of marriage, dated again, and married Marge.

He reported that although he was always emotionally and physically attracted to Marge, sex was "never great" because of her orgasm disorder.

Marge was the oldest of two sisters. She described her mother as controlling and a perfectionist. While she did not work outside the home, she ruled it with an iron first. Marge described her mother as hypercritical and that she could rarely do anything right. Marge's father was a passive man who took orders from his wife but often rebelled passive aggressively.

Marge was a popular teen, but around age 13 she was sexually abused by a neighbor. She later experienced a date rape while in college and although she was repulsed by the incident, she said that she had an orgasm solely based on the physical stimulation. Ashamed and embarrassed, she has never been able to orgasm since. Marge said that she kept the incident to herself because she did not want to upset the family. She also said that her mother would probably blame her for what had happened. She did not report the date rape because she had already slept with the man once before and worried that she would be discriminated against.

Marge noticed her orgasm issues early on and sometimes broke off with boys after one sexual encounter to prevent them from learning she had a problem. In her first marriage, she claimed that people thought that she was in control. She admitted that she was somewhat more dominant, but that her first husband was far from a push over. She claimed that he often fought back using an array of passive-aggressive tactics. She eventually decided to leave him and was matched up with Sam by a friend on a blind date.

Marge claimed that she loved Sam's direct confrontational approach compared to her former husband's style. She said Sam was a "real man." Marge agreed that sex with Sam was particularly good except for the orgasm issue. But because the disorder has lasted, she is not as interested in fixing it at this point. Prior to attending couples therapy, Marge had several years of individual therapy with a female clinician to deal with her abuse; Sam had never experienced therapy before. Let us see how Sam and Marge respond to connecting their family of origin to their control struggles in general and with sex.

Therapist: It sounds as if both of you grew up with at least one controlling parent.

Marge: My mother was ridiculous, and so was Sam's father.

Therapist: Do you agree, Sam?

Sam: Yes, my father wanted to control everything I did. If I didn't major in what he wanted me to he threatened not to pay for my tuition. I had to be an engineer.

Therapist: So, it's not a stretch to admit that the two of you are carrying on the tradition of engaging in a control struggle with each other, and with those around you.

Marge: I never thought of it that way but yes, we are both "control freaks."

Sam: But what does this have to do with our sexual problem?

Marge: I get it. Sam wants me to have more sex and to have an orgasm and I want him to stop trying to force me to do so. Given my abuse, I especially resent someone trying to force sex on me. It's like revisiting my trauma.

Therapist: Yes, to you it may be replicating your abuse but this time you are fighting back for control over your body. I certainly empathize with what you are doing, but I doubt that this style will bring authentic control to either of you. The conflict here is that both of you were controlled by one parent and disliked that aspect of them. But this parent was also the more engaged parent, who showed spunk. You both were repelled but attracted to this and you have found this same conflict in each other. Now we must see what we can do about it so that we can alleviate your control struggle over sex.

Step 5. Integrating Internal Conflict and Increasing Differentiation

Both Sam and Marge were very bright and open, but in different ways. Marge was much more insightful than Sam. In fact, she still enjoyed learning more about herself and the couple. Sam was a tougher sell, especially when offered a counterintuitive perspective. This final step in the couple's treatment differs from the previous cases presented in its need for the integration of sex therapy exercises.

Therapist: Marge, you like strong men but hate being told what to do. What are you going to do about this?

Marge: I don't know. It sounds impossible to reconcile with.

Therapist: Let's discuss the origin of this conflict. We know that you were controlled by your perfectionist mother and that's probably where your disdain for being controlled comes from; this and of course your sexual traumas. I suspect that after growing up with these experiences you now prefer to be the one in control. While this is fine, I also suspect that you take this too far. You're an adult now, not a little girl, so unless you give the oaky, you can stop most men or women who might try to dominate you. You can certainly stop Sam. But ironically, it seems to me that by overreacting to someone's control you are in a sense, acting like the powerless little girl again. You do not have to let anyone abuse you; you are in control of your body. I know it is scary to let go, but by holding onto to your victim you will limit your ability to experience sexual pleasure. And truth be told, allowing someone to take control at times can be fun. Do you really think Sam means you harm?

Marge: No, but how can I let go?

Therapist: That is what we need to continue to work on. We need to help you see your strength so that you can trust yourself and Sam. You will not feel comfortable with your current level of control by living with an angry husband. And Sam, you must help Marge to trust you. The more you try to control Marge, the more you remind her of her mother and her past traumas. To do so, you will need to stop yourself from reacting so strongly to Marge's control. You too are a capable adult. Just as your father did, you are perceiving Marge as holding the key to your masculinity. But the more you fight her, the less control you will have; she will fight you because you scare her.

Sam: I don't want to frighten Marge. I love her but I distrust that she'll work on this issue if I don't pressure her.

Marge: I'm here, aren't I?

Therapist: Well, let's see if you two are game enough to try a few exercises that might help with your orgasm disorder. I believe that we can skip Sensate Focus I & II because you are successful at foreplay and intercourse. Instead, Marge, I would like you to use your vibrator while Sam is sitting in a remote part of the same room. Focus on your feelings, not Sam's presence. Do not worry about having an orgasm—no pressure—just focus on the feeling that the vibrator creates. Try this exercise at least twice during the week and we will see how it goes. If you both agree, Marge, you can help Sam have an orgasm either manually or via oral stimulation before the exercise. But for now, refrain having intercourse.

The following week the couple tried the first exercise, but it failed because Marge insisted that Sam close his eyes while sitting in the bedroom. He refused and said it was not part of the instructions.

Therapist: So, what happened?

Sam: Marge took control and changed the exercise.

Marge: I did not. The therapist never said anything about watching me.

Therapist: Fair enough Marge. Try again this week and let Sam watch from a distance.

The couple were able to carry out the exercise and Marge achieved an orgasm while Sam sat and watched. Marge was urged to focus on her feelings and ignore Sam.

Therapist: So, what happened?

Sam: That went well.

Therapist: How were you feeling Marge?

Marge: Not bad. The orgasm was good.

Therapist: Okay, now I would like Sam to move closer and into a position you can see him.

The couple were successful again and completed the exercise twice during the week. Next, Marge was to use her vibrator while Sam was sitting on the bed next to her.

Therapist: How did it go?

Marge: It went great. At first, I was a little scared. I kept thinking Sam would jump in and take control. But he didn't. He just sat there. I had another orgasm.

Therapist: Excellent. I suspect in that fearful moment you were on the verge of regressing.

Marge: Yeah, but I now know that I can stop him.

The following exercise dictated that Sam lay next to Marge while she uses her vibrator. I knew that the closer Sam was to Marge during sexual activity, the more vulnerable and out-of-control she would feel.

Therapist: How did the exercise go this week?

Sam: Marge wanted to turn her back towards me, but I refused to cooperate, so she dropped the vibrator and left the room.

Marge: I know. I don't think I am ready for this one.

Therapist: Why not?

Marge: I felt more threatened by him laying so close to me, I guess. But I'll try again.

Marge did well this time. She was feeling her power. The therapist should expect a few detours and adjustments along the way, but as the partners learn to trust each other, and if they have faith in the therapist, the odds are good they will stay the course.

Therapist: So, what happened this week?

Marge: I did it! And I had another orgasm.

Therapist: Were you scared?

Marge: A tiny bit, but nothing like in the past.

The next exercise was for Marge to hold the vibrator on her clitoris and for Sam to gently put his hand on top of Marge's hand. He was not to guide or control her hand but to follow her movements. Thankfully, Sam controlled his need to take over.

Marge: I can't believe that worked. Well, the first time we did it I didn't have an orgasm, but I did the second time.

Therapist: That's fine.

Sam: Yeah, we are getting there. I felt like putting pressure on Marge's hand to increase her stimulation, but I held back.

Therapist: I'm glad you did.

In the next exercise, Sam was to hold the vibrator and place it on Marge's clitoris with Marge's hand was on top of his. I knew this would be a tough hurdle for the couple. Predictably, they failed to complete this exercise for two consecutive weeks.

Therapist: What happened?

Marge: I told Sam to be gentle and he shoved the vibrator on my clitoris. I thought he was too rough. I stopped the exercise because he was being pushy and abusive.

Sam: I was trying to do the exercise. I don't have as light a tough as you do.

Therapist: This is two weeks in a row with the same blockage. Sam, I suspect you're reacting to Marge's control over the intensity of the exercise. And you're fighting her.

Sam: Yeah, it's bothering me a bit. But I'll get there.

The couple finally completed this exercise. They were then to repeat the exercise, only this time Marge could turn the vibrator off whenever she felt uncomfortable. In giving her back some control, Sam was less likely to sabotage the exercise. And I was right.

Therapist: This was a big one. How did you do?

Marge: We did it. I turned the vibrator off twice just to test Sam's reactions, but he was fine.

Therapist: That's great. That was a tough one. Good job.

In the next exercise Marge was told to hold the vibrator while Sam penetrated her from a side angle. Often when intercourse is added to the exercise the therapist may experience some resistance. But not this time.

Sam: This was great. Marge and I had simultaneous orgasms.

Therapist: Any anxiety Marge?

Marge: Just a little, but I was fine.

The next exercise turned out to be the last. Marge had used a vibrator for so long that neither partner felt like forsaking the vibrator for a more natural orgasm. The final exercise was for Sam to hold the vibrator while the couple had intercourse from a side angle.

Marge: That was great. We both had orgasms. I think we're done.

Therapist: You don't want to go any further?

Sam: I'm satisfied. We were never looking for perfection.

Therapist: Okay, if you two are happy, I'm happy.

Sam desired a strong partner in Marge, but he could not tolerate her opinions and independence. To balance this internal conflict, he had to reach a compromise with these opposing parts, to better integrate them. Specifically, he would have to stop battling his tyrannical father, become less sensitive to feeling emasculated, and allow himself to be more vulnerable. Marge's sexual control and orgasmic difficulty threatened his masculinity just as his tough-guy father did. Marge had to integrate the part of her that is attractive to a tough guy and the part of her that wants to be in control. To do this she would have to forsake feeling like a powerless victim—someone who is still vulnerable to being controlled as she once was—and to own her power.

References

Abdel-Hamid, I.A., & Ali, O.I. (2018). Delayed ejaculation: Pathophysiology, diagnosis, and treatment. *World Journal of Men's Health, 36*, 22–40. https://doi.org/10.5534/wjmh.17051

American Psychiatric Association (2013). *Diagnostic and statistical manual of mental disorders* (5th ed.). https://doi.org/10.1176/appi.books.9780890425596

American Psychological Association (2020). *APA dictionary of psychology*. Retrieved August 25, 2021, from https://dictionary.apa.org/waiting-list-phenomenon

American Urological Association (2020). *Disorders of ejaculation: An AUA/SMSNA guideline*. www.auanet.org/guidelines/disorders-of-ejaculation.

Avery-Clark, C., & Weiner, L. (2018, July). *Sensate focus: The alchemy of touch, mindfulness & somatic therapy*. Training sponsored by The Integrative Sex Therapy Institute, Training Program, Washington, DC.

Betchen, S. (1997, March). *Sexual pursuer-distancer dynamics in couples therapy* [Paper presentation]. Society for Sex Therapy and Research Annual Meeting, Chicago, IL, United States.

Betchen, S. (2005). *Intrusive partner-elusive mates: The pursuer-distance dynamic in couples*. Routledge.

Betchen, S., & Davidson, H. (2018). *Master conflict therapy: A new model for practicing couples and sex therapy*. Routledge.

Betchen, S., & Gambescia, N. (2020). A new systemic treatment model for couples with premature ejaculation. In K. Hertlein, N. Gambescia, & G. Weeks (Eds.), *Systemic sex therapy* (3rd ed., pp. 77–91). Routledge.

Bhasin, S., & Basson, R. (2015). Sexual dysfunction in men and women. In S. Melmed, K.S. Polonsky, P.R. Larsen, & H. Kronenberg (Eds.), *Williams textbook of endocrinology* (13th ed., pp. 755–830). Elsevier.

Borrelli, L. (2015, April 15). *Use it or lose it: How age, hormones, and masturbation predict sexual health*. www.medicaldaily.com/use-it-or-lose-it-how-age-hormones-and-masturbation-predict-sexual-health-329366

Boszormenyi-Nagy, I., & Spark, G. (1973). *Invisible loyalties*. Harper & Row.

Briken, P., Matthiesen, S., Pietras, L., Wiessner, C., Klein, V., Reed, G., & Dekker, A. (2020). Estimating the prevalence of sexual dysfunction using the new ICD-11 guidelines: Results of the first representative, Population-Based German Health and Sexuality Survey (GeSiD). *Deutsches Arzteblatt International, 117*(39), 653–658.

Brotto, L. (2018). *Better sex through mindfulness: How women can cultivate desire*. Greystone Books.

Carvalheira, A., Traeen, B., & Štulhofer, A. (2014). Correlates of men's sexual interest: A cross-cultural study. *Journal of Sexual Medicine*, *11*, 54–164. https://doi.org/10.1111/jsm.12345. Epub 2013Oct 28

Clayton, A., & Ramamurthy, S. (2008). The impact of physical illness on sexual dysfunctions. *Advances in Psychometric Medicine*, *29*, 70–88. https://doi.org/10.1159/000126625

Corona, G., Mannucci, E., Petrone, L., Giommi, R., Fei, L., . . . Maggi, M. (2004). Psycho-biological correlates of hypoactive sexual desire in patients with erectile dysfunction. *International Journal of Impotence Research*, *16*, 275–281. https://doi.org/10.111/j1743-6109.2010.01812.x

Cultural India (2017, June 5). *Arranged marriage.* www.culturalindia.net/weddings/arranged-marriage.html

Di Sante, S., Mollaiolo, D., Gravina, G.L., Ciocca, G., & Limioncin, E. (2016). Epidemiology of delayed ejaculation. *Translational Andrology & Urology*, *5*, 541–548. https://doi.org/10.21037/tau.2016.05.10

Eplov, L., Giraldi, A., Davidsen, M., Garde, K., & Kamper-Jurgensen, F. (2007). Sexual desire in a nationally representative Danish population. *Journal of Sexual Medicine*, *4*, 47–56. https://doi.org/10.1111/j.1743-6109.2006.00396.x

Fertel, E., Meana, M., & Maykut, C. (2020). Painful intercourse: Genito-pelvic pain penetration disorder. In K. Hertlein, N. Gambescia, & G. Weeks (Eds.), *Systemic sex therapy* (3rd ed., pp. 145–159). Routledge.

Foley, S., & Gambescia, N. (2020). The complex etiology of delayed ejaculation: Assessment and treatment implications. In K. Hertlein, N. Gambescia, & G. Weeks (Eds.), *Systemic sex therapy* (3rd ed., pp. 92–106). Routledge.

Fox, D. (2020). The mind-body connection: Couples, sex, and somatic therapy. In T. Nelson (Ed.). *Integrative sex & couples therapy: A therapist's guide to new and innovative approaches* (pp. 123–133). PESI Publishing & Media.

Fugl-Meyer, A.R., & Fugl-Meyer, K.S, Fugl-Meyer, K.S., Fugl-Meyer, A.R., Sjogren, K., Fugl Meyer, K.S., Sjogren, K., & Meyer, K. (1999). Sexual disabilities, problems and satisfaction in 18–74-year-old Swedes. *Scandinavian Journal of Sexology*, *2*, 79–105.

Gambescia, N., Weeks, G., & Hertlein, K. (2021). *A clinician's guide to systemic sex therapy.* Routledge.

Gottman, J., & Silver, N. (2015). *The seven principles for making marriage work* (rev. ed.). Harmony Books.

Hall, K. (2020). Male hypoactive sexual desire disorder. In K. Hertlein, N. Gambescia, & G. Weeks (Eds.). *Systemic sex therapy* (3rd ed., pp. 41–59). Routledge.

Hall, K., & Graham, C.A. (2014). Culturally sensitive sex therapy: The need for shared meanings in the treatment of sexual problems. In Y. Binik & K.S. Hall (Eds.), *Principles and practice of sex therapy* (5th ed., pp. 334–358). Guilford Press.

Koskimäki, J., Shiri, R., Tammela, T., Häkkinen, J., Hakama, M., & Auvinen, A. (2008). Regular intercourse protects against erectile dysfunction: Tampere aging male urologic study. *The American Journal of Medicine*, *21*, 592–596. https://doi.org/10.1016/j.amjmed.2008.02.042

Lee, C. (2013). The cross-cultural encounter: Meeting the challenge of culturally competent counseling. In C. Lee (Ed.), *Multicultural issues in counseling: New approaches to diversity* (4th ed., pp. 13–19). American Counseling Association.

Lee, C., & Park, D. (2013). A conceptual framework for counseling across cultures. In C. Lee & D. Park (Eds.), *Multicultural issues in counseling: New approaches to diversity* (4th ed., pp. 3–12). American Counseling Association.

Lewis, R.W., Fugl-Meyer, K.S., Corona, G., Hayes, R.D., Laumann, E.O. Moreira, E.D., Jr., . . . Segarves, T. (2010). Definitions/epidemiology/risk factors for sexual dysfunction. *Journal of Sexual Medicine, 7,* 1598–1607. https://doi.org/10.1111/j.1743-6109.2010.01778.x

Masters, W., & Johnson, V. (1966). *Human sexual response.* Little, Brown & Company.

Masters, W., & Johnson, V. (1970). *Human sexual inadequacy.* Little, Brown & Company.

McCabe, M.P., Hertlein, K., & Davis, E. (2020). Female orgasmic disorder. In K. Hertlein, N. Gambescia, & G. Weeks (Eds.). *Systemic sex therapy* (3rd ed., pp. 130–144). Routledge.

McCarthy, B., & McCarthy, E. (2013). *Rekindling desire* (2nd ed.). Routledge.

McDaniel, S., & deGruy, F.V. (2014). An introduction to primary care and psychology. *American Psychologist, 69,* 325–331. https://doi.org/10.1037/a0036222

Meana, M., & Steiner, E.T. (2014). Hidden disorder/hidden desire: Presentations of low desire in men. In Y.M. Binik & K.S. Hall (Eds.), *Principles and practice of sex therapy* (5th ed., pp. 42–60). Guilford Press.

Metz, M., & McCarthy, B. (2007). Ejaculatory problems. In L. Vandecreek, F.L. Peterson, & J.W. Bley (Eds.), *Innovations in clinical practice: Focus on sexual Health* (pp. 115–155). Professional Resource Press.

Mintz, L. (2018). *Becoming cliterate.* HarperOne.

Nagoski, E. (2021). *Come as you are.* Simon & Schuster.

Nimbi, F.M., Ciocca, G., Limoncin, E., Fontanesi, L., Uysal, Ű.B., Flinchum, M., Tambelli, R., Jannini, E.A., & Simonelli, C. (2020). Sexual desire and fantasies in the LBGT + community: Focus on lesbian women and gay men. *Current Sexual Health Reports, 12,* 153–161. https://doi.org/doi.org/10.1007/s11930-020-00263-7

Peixoto, M.M., & Nobre, P. (2016). Personality traits, sexual problems and sexual orientations: An empirical study. *Journal of Sex and Marital Therapy, 43,* 199–213. https://doi.org/10.1080/0092623X.2014985352

Perelman, M. (2018). Why the sexual tipping point is a variable switch model? *Current Sexual Health Report, 10,* 38–43. https://doi.org/10.1007/s1193

Perelman, M. (2020). Delayed ejaculation. In K. Hall, & Y. Binik (Eds.), *Principles and practice of sex therapy* (6th ed., pp. 156–179). Guilford.

Perelman, M., & Watter, D. (2016). Delayed ejaculation. In S. Levine, C. Risen, & S. Althof (Eds.), *Handbook of clinical sexuality for mental health professionals* (3rd ed., pp. 150–162). Routledge.

Raisanen, J.C., Chadwick, S.B., Michalak, N., & van Anders, S.M. (2018). Average associations between sexual desire, testosterone, and stress in women and men over time. *Archives of Sexual Behavior, 47,* 1613–1631. https://doi.org/10.1007/s10508-018-1231-6

Rogers, G. (2019, May 11). *Delayed ejaculation.* www.healthline.com/health/delayed-ejaculation

Rowland, D.L., & Kolba, T.N. (2016). Understanding orgasmic difficulty in women. *The Journal of Sexual Medicine, 13,* 1246–1254. https://doi.org/10.1016/jjsxm.2016.05.014

Rowland, D.L., & Kolba, T.N. (2018). The burden of sexual problems: Perceived effects on men's and women's sexual problems. *The Journal of Sex Research, 55,* 226–235. https://doi.org/10.1080/00224499.20171332153

Schnarch, D. (2009). *Passionate marriage: Keeping love & intimacy alive in committed relationships.* W.W. Norton.

Semans, J. (1956). Premature ejaculation: A new approach. *Southern Medical Journal, 49,* 353–358.

Waelder, R. (1960). *Basic theory of psychoanalysis.* International Universities Press.

Weeks, G.R., & Gambescia, N. (2015). Definition, etiology, and treatment of absent/low desire in women. In K. Hertlein, G. Weeks, & N. Gambescia (Eds.), *Systemic sex therapy*. Routlege.

Weiner, L., & Avery-Clark, C. (2014). *Sensate focus in sex therapy*. Routledge.

Woo, J.S.T., Morshedian, N., Brotto, L.A., & Gorzalka, B.B. (2012). Sex guilt mediates the relationship between religiosity and sexual desire in East Asians and Euro-Canadian college-aged women. *Archives of Sexual Behavior, 41,* 1485–1495. https://doi.org/10.1007/s10508-012-9918-6

7   How the Couples Therapist Can Avoid Being Caught in a Control Struggle

If the couples therapist encounters a particularly controlling couple, their struggle will bleed into the therapeutic process. To avoid being paralyzed by this process or rendered clinically impotent, the therapist must remember that although both partners may act as if they want control, there also exists a part in each that prefers to be out-of-control. Blocking the therapist from resolving their internal conflict serves to maintain this conflict and in turn, prevent the pain that comes with change. To further achieve this objective, the couple will inadvertently try to trap the therapist so that change is difficult if not impossible. But the therapist is not helpless. There are myriad techniques that can be used to avoid this trap.

Joining

One way to prevent getting caught in a control struggle with a couple is to appropriately "join" with them early in the therapeutic process (Minuchin, 1974) and to continue to do so throughout treatment (Colapinto, 1982). But because couples therapy is considered the hardest therapy (Doherty, 2002), this is no easy task. In individual treatment the therapist must join with one person. But in couples therapy, the therapist must join with two partners who usually do not agree on a variety of issues—sometimes even the chief complaint.

Joining is considered by some systems therapists to be a form of empathy (Minuchin, 1974) and some psychoanalysts are close to agreeing with this. Kohut (1979), for example, defined empathy as a form of "vicarious introspection." Having shared experiences might evoke a certain empathy and in turn, greatly enhance the joining process. For example, if partners and therapist shared similar losses, it might be easier for all parties to relate.

It is also easier for the therapist to join with a couple if they all share similar interests. For example, perhaps they play the same musical instrument, or share a love of foreign film. Maybe they are both handy around the house or can fix cars. This does not necessarily mean that the therapist must divulge personal information. Just showing a sincere interest implies a connection with the couple and will often suffice. But because this is not a matter of the end justifying the means, a couple should never be lied to for the sake of joining. If the couple were originally from Utah, for example, do not tell them that you once lived

DOI: 10.4324/9781003159100-10

there if it is not true. Do not tell them you come from a big family if you are an only child. Simply put, do not fabricate a story; it is not worth the risk. If you are caught lying you will have destroyed the couple's trust in you, and most likely cause irreparable damage to the treatment process.

Telling the truth, however, does not mean that some information might be better withheld for the good of the relationship. For example, a female client called to request marital therapy. She admitted that she had an affair but ended it and wanted to work on her marriage. I hesitated to take the case because her husband did not know about the affair, and I assumed that he might be upset with me if he ever found out that I did. But rather than struggle with the woman, I decided to take a chance for four reasons: (1) the affair was apparently over, and the wife seemed sincere in her desire to work on her marriage; (2) because I felt bound by confidentiality to the wife, I felt justified in taking the risk; (3) the wife was remorseful that she had acted in a deceitful manner; and (4) the couple had small children. The husband did eventually find out about the affair—his wife confessed in a moment of guilt—and I had to then rebuild his trust in me. Luckily, he gave both of us another chance after I explained that if he were in the same position as his wife, I would have had to keep his confidentiality as well.

Some therapists may find it valuable to mimic certain mannerisms of the client to join such as copying a hand gesture or crossing legs a certain way (Minuchin, 1993). I too, have on occasion dressed somewhat differently to accommodate certain clients. For example, I might dress conservatively knowing that a couple will feel more at ease. But on the rare occasion that a couples therapist cannot find anything that can be used to relate to the couple, it might help to simply give them credit for being brave enough to enter treatment and expose their innermost secrets.

In some cases, one or both partners may be overly sensitive, and if wounded may join against the therapist. This can be both good and bad. It is good when partners agree, but under these conditions they may be inclined to gang up on the couple's therapist and try to take control of the treatment by way of intimidation. When a therapist faces this challenge, it might be helpful to confront the joint resistance and interpret it to the couple as potentially sabotaging to the treatment.

Escaping a Double Bind

Sometimes a controlling couple will inadvertently place the therapist in a dilemma that many refer to as a double bind—a concept once thought to be the cause of schizophrenia (Bateson et al., 1956). In a double bind, one partner might make a request of the therapist and yet punish the therapist for acquiescing. These messages may be stated or implicit in the context of a relationship. Paradoxical in nature, this can be quite confusing to the therapist and make it impossible to please the couple.

The double bind is known in popular culture as a catch-22 (Heller, 2011) or a "damned if you do, and damned if you don't" situation. For example, one or both partners may pressure you to provide specific interventions or to be more active in the treatment. But when you do become more assertive, they may constantly interrupt you or disagree with everything you say. Some couples may request the impossible of you and yet become upset when you cannot meet their demands. The following brief exchange illustrates this dynamic with the husband of a couple:

Hank: (To the therapist) Doctor, aren't you going to say something? I'm paying for this, and I think you need to earn your pay.

Therapist: You're asking me what I think about your boss, but I don't know him. I only know what you tell me. But I do think you might be having a control struggle with him . . .

Hank: (Interrupts) That's ridiculous. Is that all you have to say?

Therapist: So, you reject my . . .

Hank: (Interrupts) I disagree with you, and I think with your training you should be able to come up with something a little deeper.

There are several ways that a couples therapist can handle a catch-22. The first is to gently but directly address the double bind: "I really want to help you, but I feel as if you have me in a bind: No matter what I say to you, it will not suffice. Can you help me out here so that I can be of some service to you?" This response puts the responsibility for the double bind directly back on the couple. If this tactic fails, I might ask the couple: "How can I help you? What do you want to hear from me?" This is even more challenging because it forces the couple to come up with a solution to the bind that they have placed you in. If these tactics fail, as they did with Hank, I may get a little more assertive. For example, I eventually had to say to him: "You seem to have better ideas than I have, so let's talk about how you think you should handle your colleagues." I also told a couple: "If you render me helpless, there may be no hope for any of us."

If all else fails, I may refer the couple to a different therapist. But in doing so, I never predict failure for the couple. I prefer to let the couple know that in therapy the "fit" between the couple and the couple's therapist is most important, and that it is natural that they might not feel a fit with me. I never suggest that the couple are not for me—that might be taken as an insult and evoke a control struggle in and of itself. I also never imply that I am the best or only therapist that can help them. I usually tell the couple that they might work better with someone else, and that there are plenty of therapists out there who may do a better job with them than I can. At a couple's request, I will even do my best to offer appropriate referrals. There is no need to get in a struggle at this point just to prove you are right. There will be no winner in this contest. If the therapist wishes to avoid a control struggle, this can be achieved most of the time. But if the therapist is looking for a fight or to prove oneself, a struggle can be found. I would, however, warn the therapist to be careful what is wished for.

In less complex situations, a more disarming way to avoid being caught in a catch-22 is available. That is, if I sense that the couple can take a joke, I might use humor. I once said to a husband who pressured me to cure his premature ejaculation but admitted that he lacked the patience for sex therapy exercises: "I think you are pulling out too early again." I also might use humility: For example, "You two are much smarter than I am so I'm going to need your help figuring out how to solve a puzzle that may be difficult to solve." When it comes to escaping a couple's attempt to control the treatment, the therapist must use instinct and impeccable timing all while maintaining dyadic balance.

Intuition and Timing

According to Shallcross (2016), intuition "is something that is known or understood without proof or evidence" (p. 1). Fox (2013) found that many counselors credited their intuition as being more influential in their work than evidence-based treatments. Therapists tend to be sensitive beings who are attuned to an individual's vulnerability. I believe this comes naturally to them because most innately possess these traits and tendencies. This is no different than an individual who is better with things than people being drawn to the field of engineering.

Most therapists can tell when to challenge a defense and when to wait. They know to be careful when confronting an angry couple, or a couple who insist on perceiving themselves as victims. Most therapists know better than to joke with a humorless client, or one who may be too depressed to appreciate lightness. Couples therapists are also skilled at telling which partner is more, or less, committed to treatment. They know that challenging or engaging in a struggle or challenging the initiator of treatment may end in the ultimate act of control: premature termination. Simply put, mistakes in this area might result in losing control over the therapeutic process.

Unilateral Aligning Versus Balancing

Balancing multiple alliances is most valuable in couples therapy whereas split alliances can be problematic (Friedlander et al., 2018). It is far easier to get caught in a control struggle if you make the mistake of aligning with one partner of a couple. Once you do that, you join forces against the other mate. That mate in turn, will most likely feel provoked enough to do battle with you. Even if you miraculously avoid being fired by this mate—who will feel betrayed and disappointed—you will be contaminating the treatment by reinforcing or exacerbating the couple's internal conflict around control. If this occurs, there will be little hope of you helping the couple to balance their conflict.

There are numerous balancing techniques that can be used to avoid aligning with a partner. For example, I take turns looking at each partner throughout the treatment even when only one is speaking, I continuously shift my eyes from one to the other. It is a subtle way of including both partners in every aspect of the treatment process, giving the couple the impression that I take no sides. Another technique I use is to ask one partner to comment on what the other has said. Again, the objective is to maintain balance so that I do not appear to take sides. I also take turns complimenting each partner for his/her input: "That is an important point, and I am glad you were here to help." Even if I think a partner is making an irrational comment I will lead with: "I get your point . . .," before I challenge the comment.

Last, I always try to find at least one thing in each partner that I admire or respect . . . and hold onto it throughout the treatment. It could be something I admire such as a financial or emotional feat of some kind. For example, although a male client's narcissism has apparently alienated many people in his life, he held my respect because I believed him to be a financial genius. A middle-aged female client had a gruff disposition which was on the verge of costing her a marriage. But while most people avoided her, I respected the fact that she was a self-made woman who had survived many traumas in her life. And a male client who was especially oppositional had the knowledge and skills to build his own home. I would not even know where to start such a project. To soften a particularly difficult or controlling client I locate this area of admiration or respect and I acknowledge it. I believe that it is important to give credit where credit is due no matter how the therapist may feel about the overall personality of the client.

Setting Boundaries

Boundaries have long been an important concept in all of psychotherapy, and in particular, systems treatment where there is more opportunity to breach them (Minuchin & Fishman, 1981). And they are especially vital in maintaining control over the therapeutic process. Perhaps more than any other mishap, failure to set and maintain boundaries can further imbalance a couple's conflict and result in greater chaos.

Just as with any other concept, boundary issues exist on a continuum with a severe breach on one end and a mild, relatively harmless breach on the other. In taking a class for certification as a clinical supervisor, the question was posed by the instructor about the harm that can be done if a therapist has sex with a client. While there was a consensus that this was inappropriate behavior on the part of the therapist—and I agreed—I raised my hand and added another perspective: "I wouldn't want to give a client that much control over me." The room went silent, but my point was simply that it was not only harmful to the client involved but the therapist as well. While the client might suffer from the aftereffects of such a relationship, the therapist could lose control over his/her reputation and livelihood. What might start out feeling like control may end in both parties being out-of-control. The same would apply to going into business with a client. Any boundary breach in the therapeutic environment which could end up in disciplinary action or sabotage the couple's treatment process is not worth the risk. It is the stuff that makes it difficult for therapists to sleep at night.

Linn (2019) advocates establishing rules in the treatment process, but some couples try their hardest to break them, and some therapists enable them to do so. Couples therapy commands little control over a couple. All the couple is asked to do is to show up for scheduled appointments and pay their fees. It would be nice if they engaged in the treatment process, but that is up to them—it will depend on how much they want to improve their plight. Nevertheless, therapists routinely struggle with collecting and raising fees, ending sessions on time, and charging for cancellations. Rules lead to structure and help a couple to balance a *control versus out-of-control* conflict. Couples do not need to see a therapist who is out-of-control; this would be a poor role model for clients who are trying to make some sense out of their chaos.

When it comes to rule breaking, couples therapy offers many subtle opportunities for partners to take advantage of process and in turn, further unbalance their internal conflict with control. Supervisees, for example, have asked me how I would handle a partner who might linger in my office after a session just to get a few extra jabs in about his/her counterpart; or the partner who calls or emails without their respective partner's knowledge. Many therapists do not relish going over the rules of treatment with clients before they feel they have joined with them. Others put these rules in writing and give them to the couple before the first session. While these ideas are important to consider, boundary crossing is often an unconscious process, and couples sometimes employ them unaware of the damage they might be doing. This makes sense given that their internal conflict is beyond their level of awareness. If a breach occurs after the rules of treatment are set, my recommendation would be to politely re-explain the general rules and to perhaps get more specific. In this case, I would simply tell the partner that communicating with me without their partner's knowledge could anger their counterpart, unbalance the treatment, and end in premature termination. I would not tell the counterpart what the other is doing, but if the behavior continues, after a warning I would discuss termination and a referral with the breaching partner. It would then be up to him/her whether to confess or not. I would frame it as: "Couples therapy does not seem merited at this point in time."

Some partners try to control treatment by requesting individual sessions. I will only offer these for the following reasons: (1) if I suspect that a partner is not invested in the treatment because of an affair or for some other potentially destructive reason; (2) if a partner is stuck on a particular issue that merits a more intense look at the family of origin to catch up to the other partner; and (3) if I suspect there was something that I need to know that is too difficult or embarrassing to talk about in front of the partner, such as sexual abuse. If I do see a partner individually I usually only do so for no more than five sessions to preserve the systemic integrity of the treatment process. For balance, I will also request that the other partner follow by having the same number of individual sessions (Berman, 1982; Weeks et al., 2005).

The Therapist's Conflict With Control

Whether we speak of "countertransference" (Freud, 1910/1957), "the therapist use of the self" (Satir, 2000), or "the person of the therapist" (Aponte & Kissil, 2016), we are referring to the reaction of the therapist to clients in the therapeutic environment. In MCT (Betchen & Davidson, 2018), it is important that the couples therapist be aware of his/her internal conflict to effectively work with couples. As mentioned, partners who form long-term relationships share the same conflict; they unconsciously choose each other for this very reason. While it is not known whether a couple and therapist do the same, I have found that if couple and therapist do share the same conflict, an instant relationship will form, bonding between couple and therapist will be easier, and the therapist should have little trouble empathizing with his/her theoretical twins. The therapist will also find a couple with a similar conflict more interesting. But if the therapist has not sufficiently integrated his/her conflict—even if they are the same—it will be much more difficult to help the couple to do so.

With regards to the *control versus out-of-control* conflict, the therapist is likely to mimic the couple's behavior and vacillate between being in and out-of-control. This may manifest in intermittent diffuse boundaries, limit-setting problems, and therapeutic chaos. There will be some structure and control, but chaos will follow because of the simultaneous need to lose control. Simply put, the treatment will be less stable if the therapist enables the couple to gain and lose control over their relationship and their lives. Some examples that come to mind are: (1) the couples therapist is often late to the sessions—if this is a chronic problem, the couple will soon mimic this behavior without fearing any consequences, especially if they are still given a full session. One couple said to a supervisee: "You're late, why can't we be?" I argued that the couple had a point. If the supervisee is upset by their lateness, one way to fix this would be to call it even and to no longer role model lateness; (2) the couples therapist allows sessions to run over several minutes. If there is a crisis, like a partner just discovered a mate's affair in the waning minutes of a session, it is hard to ask a couple to leave your office before settling them down or making an immediate referral. But if this becomes a pattern, the couple will get used to the lack of structure and feel entitled to more time.

A highly disorganized couple with terrible limit-setting issues inadvertently mentioned that their previous couples therapist would often see them for up to three hours at any one time even though they were officially scheduled for a 55-minute-session. This not only fed into the couple's pathology, but inconvenienced couples that followed; (3) being inconsistent with your fee structure such as charging too little or too much for your services. Most therapists will adjust their fees downward either prior to or during treatment for a couple that demonstrates a legitimate need. Others might settle on a reduced fee because they find a particular case interesting or unusual, or because they might need hours towards a license or certification. Still others may give clients a break because they no longer have insurance through no fault of their own, or because they have suffered a financial setback that was beyond their control.

It is important to know whether the couple is dedicated to treatment or trying to further enlist the couple's therapist into their pathology. The fee itself is often the context for this dynamic. For example, a couple requested a substantial fee reduction from one of my colleagues; despite solid professional credentials, both were underachieving financially. They neglected to complete their professional licensures and preferred to work less than full-time; there was also a history of victimization. Because of these factors, my colleague decided to offer a reasonably reduced rate—but higher than the fee proposed by the couple—that would conceivably allow the couple to continue treatment. The fee offered by the therapist did not enable the couple's victimization, and it was satisfactory to the therapist.

Charging too much for therapeutic services, especially to those that cannot afford it, will result in therapeutic chaos, and contribute to a couple feeling out-of-control. For example, a couple seriously considering divorce were referred to me by the wife's attorney in a final attempt to save the marriage. But the couple were in such dire financial straits they could not afford me even at a reduced rate. Even if they were able to stay for a few sessions I worried that they would grow further in debt and not be able to complete treatment anyway. With these concerns in mind, I told the lawyer—with the couple's permission—that the couple would be better served in a clinic that charged on a sliding scale. I told him that I was worried about feeding into their financial issues, and that he should be as well. The lawyer claimed that an insurance policy would pay and that he would take his fee out of the settlement. He wanted me to do the same. But there was no guarantee of this, and the couple could use that money for other things given their dire financial state. I again requested that the lawyer offer the couple a more appropriate referral and he finally agreed.

If the therapist is in and out-of-control in his/her personal life, it will eventually show up in the office and influence the couple's work. This may also be evident in the way interventions are delivered in treatment. The couples therapist may fail to recognize or challenge a couple when they are out-of-control or about to do something that may result in a lack of control. Here is an example: John made a good living as an attorney, but his wife Renee claimed that he took risks at his law firm that have gotten him in trouble from time to time.

Renee: John had a good year at work, but he really takes some chances.

Therapist: Can you give me an example?

Renee: Well, generally his clients like him but he has been warned to give them a running tally of their charges rather than hit them with one huge bill at the end of his work. They tend to hate that, and some have threatened never to use him again. They've even called the chairman of his firm to report him.

Therapist: Well, when you're in the service industry people are going to be dissatisfied with you from time to time—it's part of the job.

John: I told you Renee. It's no big deal. You're worrying too much.

In this example the therapist discounted the couple's conflict in rendering an intervention. This only served to enable John, and it failed to gain any favor with Renee, who was anxious. The following is a more appropriate response in MCT:

Renee: John had a good year at work, but he really took some chances.

Therapist: Can you give me an example?

Renee: Well, generally his clients like him but he has been warned to give them a running tally on their bills rather than hit them with one huge statement at the end of his work. They tend to hate that, and some have threatened never to use him again. He also rarely calls them back in a timely fashion and can be short-tempered. Some have even called the chairman of his firm to report him.

Therapist: So, John, you seem to be playing games with your conflict. That can be dangerous. One day you're in control and the next . . .

John: I'm in control. There's nothing to worry about.

Therapist: We shall see. Life is a far harsher teacher than I am, and so is the conflict.

Renee: John scares me. We need his job to survive. Can't you get through to him?

Although the therapist is free to challenge clients, it does not mean they will listen. The conflict is for the most part unconscious, and it puts up a fierce battle against change. John, for example, did not listen, and was eventually called in again by his boss and put on probation. It turns out that colleagues complained about him. But Renee played the powerless enabler—her contribution to the perpetuation of their shared control conflict. She complained about John, but failed to do enough to stop him. John was tough, but desperate times called for desperate measures. John was out-of-control at work and threatening the family's livelihood. In the following exchange, Renee is confronted:

Therapist: I understand why you are anxious Renee. Part of John's conflict calls for a loss of control. But I suspect that you have more power over this than I do.

Renee: He doesn't listen to anybody. If he won't listen to you or his boss what makes you think he'll listen to me?

Therapist: It sounds as if you are feeling out-of-control.

Renee: I'm worried.

Therapist: I know, but I am questioning your powerlessness.

Renee: What should I do?

Therapist: That sounds like the question from a woman who is feeling out-of-control. Do you want more control over your situation or don't you?

Renee: I do.

Therapist: Then I'm sure you will think of something.

Notice the therapist does not give Renee the answer. To do so might have hindered her growth and unbalanced the couple in part, because John would not have appreciated the therapist teaching Renee how to threaten him. The therapist must always keep in mind that he/she is an outsider. Couples who share a conflict have a common goal—to maintain their conflict. The therapist must be careful not to split the couple or risk being fired or accused of ending a relationship. This was Renee's risk to take.

In MCT, the couples therapist would do best to get his/her conflict balanced and under control. This can be accomplished by seeking help from a supervisor or therapist partial to a conflict perspective. Because of the systems component in treating couples, someone with both systemic and conflict theory training would be ideal, but not necessarily easy to find given the divergent philosophies of psychoanalysis and systems theory.

References

Aponte, H., & Kissil, K. (2016). *The person of the therapist training model: Mastering the use of self.* Routledge.

Bateson, G., Jackson, D., Haley, J., & Weakland, J. (1956). Toward a theory of schizophrenia. *Behavioral Science, 1,* 251–264. https://doi.org/10.1002/bs.3830010402

Berman, E. (1982). The individual interview as a treatment technique in conjoint therapy. *The American Journal of Family Therapy, 10,* 27–37. https://doi.org/10.1080/01926188208250434

Betchen, S., & Davidson, H. (2018). *Master conflict therapy: A new model for practicing couples and sex therapy.* Routledge.

Colapinto, J. (1982). Structural family therapy. In A.M. Horne & M.M. Ohlsen (Eds.), *Family counseling and therapy* (pp. 112–140). F.E. Peacock Publishers.

Doherty, W. (2002). Bad couples therapy: How to avoid doing it. *Psychotherapy Networker, 26,* 26–33.

Fox, J. (2013). *The development of the counselor intuition scale* (Publication No. 2004-2019.2626) [Doctoral dissertation, University of Central Florida]. PQDT Open. https://stars.library.ucf.edu/etd/2626

Freud, S. (1910/1957). The future prospects of psycho-analytic therapy. In J. Strachey (Ed. and Trans.), *The standard edition of the complete psychological works of Sigmund Freud* (Vol. 11, pp. 139–151). Hogarth Press and the Institute of Psycho-analysis.

Friedlander, M.L., Escudero, V., Welmers van de Poll, M.J., & Heatherington, L. (2018). Meta-analysis of the alliance-outcome relation in couples and family therapy. *Psychotherapy, 55,* 367–371. https://doi.org/10/1037/pst0000161

Heller, J. (2011). *Catch-22: Fiftieth anniversary edition.* Simon & Schuster.

Kohut, H. (1979). The two analyses of Mr. Z. *International Journal of Psycho-Analysis, 60,* 3–27.

Linn, A. (2019, August 22). *How to set boundaries with clients in a therapeutic setting: A guide for new therapists.* Allie Linn. https://medium.com/@allielinn20/how-to-set-boundaries-with-clients-in-a-therapeutic-setting-a-guide-for-new-therapists-a35f7468ccd5

Minuchin, S. (1974). *Families & family therapy*. Harvard University Press.

Minuchin, S. (1993). On family therapy. *Psychology Today, 26*, 20–23.

Minuchin, S., & Fishman, C.H. (1981). *Family therapy techniques*. Harvard University Press.

Satir, V. (2000). The therapist story. In M. Baldwin (Ed.), *The use of self in therapy* (2nd ed., pp. 17–27). Haworth.

Shallcross, L. (2016, July 24). *Embracing intuition: Counseling today*. Counseling Today. https://ct.counseling.org/2016/07/embracing-intuition/

Weeks, G., Odell, M., & Methven, S. (2005). *If only I had known . . . avoiding common mistakes in couples therapy*. W.W. Norton.

8 Termination and Relapse Prevention

Criteria for Termination

Termination of treatment is generally agreed upon by both the therapist and couple. This usually occurs when the couple has reached their stated therapeutic goals or their symptoms have dissipated enough to satisfy them (Patterson et al., 2018). In MCT, however, other criteria must be satisfied before a case is declared a success. They are as follows:

- *Both partners must realize that they share a master conflict around control that is behind their symptoms*: Without this acknowledgement, a couple will find it difficult to maintain empathy and to continue to work together to challenge their internal conflict. It will also be too easy for them to find themselves in another debilitating control struggle.
- *Both partners must accept the power of their master conflict*: Couples must respect their conflict. They must not underestimate it, or they will suffer the consequences. I warn clients that these conflicts often organically strike when the clients are feeling at their best because the conflict never completely dissipates.
- *Both partners must realize that they are prone to control struggles in other contexts beyond the one they presented as the chief complaint*: This is a common cause of recidivism. I have had numerous couples terminate their therapy successfully only to return because they were having trouble in a different context such as at work or with friends. They are often quite surprised to find that while their content or context changed, their process or master conflict is the same.
- *Both partners understand where their respective control struggles have originated from*: Ahistorical therapists do not necessarily agree with this, but as a psychodynamic couples therapist I believe that understanding the origin of a conflict is important. First it validates the *multigenerational transmission process* (Bowen, 1978). And if nothing else, partners learn that they were not born with a tendency for control; they are products of their upbringings and life experiences.
- *Both partners understand that there is no cure for an internalized master conflict*: It is relieving for a couple to re-experience their conflict without

DOI: 10.4324/9781003159100-11

feeling like a failure. I even warn them to expect that their conflict "will" cause them future difficulty. Those that do well come to view their conflict like an ornery family member whose nature it is to flare up from time to time.

• *Both partners realize that the best they can do with an internal master conflict is to learn how to manage it . . . and this will be good enough*: Couples are relieved when they hear that they only need to work towards managing their conflict rather than changing their entire beings to alleviate their symptoms. It is far less daunting to think in terms of a therapeutic adjustment rather than perfection.

• *Symptoms are alleviated to all participant's satisfaction*: This will be discussed later in greater detail, but it is best if both the couple and the therapist agree when to end treatment. This helps to prevent premature termination and recidivism.

• *The couple demonstrates fewer control struggles*: This is where the couple validates their success to themselves and to the therapist. If they clearly show that their control struggles are less frequent, it is a good indication that they are ready for termination.

• *The couple demonstrates an ability to quell a control struggle before it escalates*: Every couple will re-experience post-therapeutic control struggles. But when a couple is ready to terminate, whatever control struggles they do have are less intense, and the couple can get out of them much quicker and easier than they could in the past.

Achieving these objectives can be a formidable task which will take great commitment from the couple. While a couple is struggling to balance or rebalance their internal conflict, the couple's therapist needs to be empathic about the difficulty of this task. My experience in classical psychoanalysis has taught me that deep change is hard. To change at this level—at the level MCT demands—most people will have to be in significant pain. They will have to reach the conclusion that their symptoms and the pain they are causing are worth the price they will have to pay to change. They must be "all in" on the treatment process to succeed. I will ask a couple: "Have you ever heard anybody say that they will give medical school a try?" Although this question usually brings a chuckle from the couple, they get the message: no pain, no gain.

Normal termination is a gradual process in MCT. I see couples on a weekly basis but when terminating, I negotiate a plan with the couple. I rarely push a couple out of treatment if they are not ready, especially if they have been in treatment with me for some time. I only do so if a referral to another therapist is merited. I recommend that the couple's therapist space their final sessions out (Patterson et al., 2018). I will usually start by recommending bi-weekly sessions but allow the couple to determine how slowly we move from there. Extra time allows the couple to test their control over their conflict and to see if new symptoms develop—which is an indication that the conflict is still too out-of-control or unbalanced (Betchen & Davidson, 2018). This gradual process will also give the couple's therapist time to go over the couple's therapeutic gains (Morrill & Córdova, 2010).

Why Couples Terminate Prematurely

Premature or early termination is formally defined as dropping out of treatment before therapeutic goals are reached regardless of the number of sessions. If an agreed upon number of sessions are terminated early, it would also be considered premature termination (Bartle-Haring et al., 2012; Doss et al., 2011). Research has indicated that premature termination is a clear impediment to client improvement (Swift et al., 2018). But approximately one in every five clients end treatment prior to its conclusion (Swift & Greenberg, 2012). According to Siegel (2010), some couples find the therapeutic process, especially deep couples work, too difficult to continue. There are several reasons for this:

- *There is a problem bonding with the therapist*: Like any relationship, if couple and therapist cannot bond the relationship will be short-lived (Jurek et al., 2014). Björk et al. (2009) found premature terminators to be less satisfied with their therapist's ability to listen and to understand them. And this dissatisfaction is usually evident early on in treatment. The parties may appear agitated with one another, demonstrate difficulty communicating clearly and effectively, fail to appreciate one another's sense of humor, and disagree with one another's core values.
- *The couple may never have been committed to their relationship*: Some people treat their relationship as if it is a research experiment. They know on some level they are not willing to do what it requires to be successful. One woman told me that as she aged, she felt odd being single—she felt that people were looking at her as if she were "weird." She said that at least if she were divorced nobody would question her. Her marriage lasted a total of two years—just long enough to have a child and get out. A second example is that of a man who told me that he was never attracted to his wife. He admitted that he stayed unattached for as long as he could but finally married because he could no longer "stand being lonely." Committing to someone under these or similar circumstances usually results in a poor prognosis for the relationship.
- *The couple may have never been committed to the treatment*: Couples who report to treatment infrequently, cancel often, or make scheduling or rescheduling appointments a chore may be demonstrating therapeutic ambivalence. Here is a recent example that began with the initial telephone call:

Gayle: Hi, I would like to schedule an appointment for my husband and me. I was referred to you by two different people.

Therapist: Okay, when do you two have time?

Gayle: Well, my husband has a difficult schedule so it will have to be evenings.

Therapist: Okay, I have a 6 pm or 7 pm this Tuesday or the same next Tuesday, Wednesday, or Thursday.

Gayle: Well, we can't do Tuesdays.

Therapist: Okay, what about Wednesdays or Thursdays?

Gayle: Well, I think they may be okay, but I'll have to check my calendar and talk to my husband. Can we make an appointment two months out?

Therapist: Is your husband okay with this?

Gayle: I think so.

Therapist: (Skeptical about the couple's ability to commit to treatment) I don't schedule that far in advance. Why don't you talk to your husband, make a list of the dates and times you both can agree to, and get back to me. I'll do my best to accommodate you.

My initial impression was that the odds on this couple following through were close to zero. Although they did get back to me, after approximately two consecutive sessions, they could not agree on future times, cancelled several sessions even when they did agree on when to meet, and eventually disappeared. I tried to discuss their ambivalence, but they were not interested in processing it. Other reasons for premature termination include:

- *To avoid responsibility*: I have seen several couples drop out of therapy prematurely when they are about to be challenged. If allowed to remain on the offensive, or if their defenses are holding up, they may stay. But if either partner feels too vulnerable, he/she may find a quick way out of treatment— usually under the guise that they are mad at each other, or the therapist.
- *Because of intense anxiety*: Therapy often scares people, and a couple's format can be even more frightening because your partner is usually taking you to task. One woman dropped out prematurely because she was too frightened to deal with her sexual arousal disorder. It was connected to her sexual abuse as a child and she did not want anybody to know this, particularly her husband. She was concerned that he would see her as "damaged goods" and leave her.
- *To provoke an ending to the relationship*: A male client confessed that he married his girlfriend because he could not bear the guilt of breaking up with her. By opting out of couples therapy against her wishes, he provoked her to divorce him. Another man dropped out because he was having an affair and was not interested in improving his marriage. He did not want therapy to interfere with his affair.
- *To maintain their conflict around control*: According to Tartakovsky (2016), relationships inside the office tend to mirror relationships outside the office. By ending treatment prematurely, the couple will take control of the therapeutic process and most likely fail to resolve their conflict. The following is an example of a wife who dropped out of treatment just before

partner sessions were prescribed for her husband's premature ejaculation (PE). By doing so, she was able to: avoid being vulnerable to the therapeutic process; avoid taking any responsibility for her contributions to the couple's issues; and continue enabling the couple's control conflict.

Lena: I've had it. I'm out of here.

Therapist: But Lena, I thought you've been waiting a long time for Rick to get help. Why are you dropping out now?

Lena: Because I've waited long enough. It's his problem . . . let him show me he cares enough to fix it.

Rick: I know it took me a long time to get here but I was too embarrassed to go to the doctor.

Lena: Well, how do you think I felt?

Therapist: I understand why you're angry Lena. Rick did procrastinate. But if the bottom line is to fix your problem, he is here now.

Lena: Forget about it. I'm too angry to even try. This is a good test for him.

Therapist: It looks like you two take turns trying to be in control.

Lena: Why not? Let Rick feel what it's like to be controlled.

Therapist: But if you agree that Rick was in control at one time and now you are, aren't you doing the same thing he once did: paralyzing the process? I say this because you're important to the treatment.

Both partners may agree to terminate and if I agree with their decision, I will praise them and wish them well. Ending on good terms can teach the couple how to mimic this behavior in their relationship outside the office as well. In their best interests, however, I remind them: (1) the control conflict will always live within them; (2) as soon as they experience tension in the relationship, their control struggle should be considered first and foremost; (3) the struggle for control will show itself in other contexts but this is normal, and they now have the tools to handle it; and (4) I will be there for them if they should need me at a later date.

If I disagree with the couple's decision to terminate, I will let them know. I will immediately link the concept of premature termination to the couple's conflict and show them how it may only perpetuate their control struggle and that their symptoms are likely to reappear (Cummings, 2008; Greenan, 2010). I believe it is the job of the therapist to at least warn the couple of the potential consequences of their decision, but I resist getting into a control struggle over termination. If a couple wants to end therapy, I will not fight them. If they made a mistake, hopefully they will discover this on their own and eventually return to treatment—if not with me, then with someone else. Angering or pressuring a couple is unprofessional and will only leave a bad impression. The following is an example:

Gary: Trudi and I think we're ready to end treatment. And my sexual desire is back.

Therapist: I believe that you two have done a great job, but I wouldn't be doing my job if I didn't express some concern. While it's true that your sex drive is back, you both still disagree on the frequency of sex. To me, this is a sign that the battle for control is still somewhat significant. Perhaps you could commit to a few more sessions to work this through.

Trudi: We understand your concern, but we have discussed it thoroughly and we would like to try to work the rest out ourselves.

Therapist: Okay, if you've made up your minds, you know where to find me if you need me.

When One Partner Terminates Prematurely

Jurek et al. (2014) wrote: "A good working alliance exists when both partners are involved in the therapeutic process in an active manner and perceive it as a tool for solving their problems" (p. 55). One partner will not be able to resolve a shared conflict alone; this would be inconsistent with a systemic approach such as MCT.

In MCT, if only one partner works on his/her conflict, the other will fight vigorously to keep it at full strength, which will eventually result in an escalation of symptoms. In fact, couples are most likely to split when only one partner owns the conflict. When this occurs, the partner resistant to change may look for a replacement partner to share the conflict. To avoid this, each partner must come to believe in MCT. They must also be willing to work together towards a common therapeutic goal of managing their conflict, especially one as formidable as a conflict over control. In this situation, the therapist should immediately connect the idea of premature termination to the couple's conflict and alert the couple as to how this may only increase their control struggle and associated symptoms.

If one partner does prematurely terminate, I generally do not recommend that the couples therapist continue treatment. Given the importance of balance in couple's work, it will be far too easy to lose objectivity and become engaged in a control struggle with the absent partner. It might also lead to some ethical or legal implications for the therapist, particularly if the couple separate and the partner who dropped out accuses the therapist of ruining the relationship.

Wachtel (2017) frowns upon seeing one partner after couples therapy is terminated. It is best to tell the partner that you should remain the couple's therapist in case the couple needs help in the future. If the therapist is pressed, he/she can claim that it would imbalance the treatment and possibly sabotage everything the couple has already worked for. While many therapists will not heed these words, they should at least: (1) only agree if the couple's therapy was brief (e.g., two sessions or less); (2) get permission from the absent partner before conducting individual therapy; (3) make sure to advise both partners, especially the absent one, of the risks involved when doing individual treatment for relationship issues (Heitler, 2013); and (4) work with the abandoned partner, if possible.

Working with the abandoned partner will prove safer because this person is less likely to accuse you of destroying the relationship. It is even safer to avoid treating the individual until a divorce is finalized, but this is not always practical, in part, because the individual may require immediate help or because many couples linger. Consider the following scenario involving a Hispanic couple seen for two sessions:

Mateo: I'm out of here. I can't do this anymore. I only tried out of respect for Mariana. But I want a divorce.

Mariana: Some try. I hope you didn't strain yourself.

Mateo: See, she's so hostile. This is one of the major reasons I want to leave. I think she needs your help doc.

Mariana: If he wants to leave, he can leave, but I would like to stay on. I think you and I get along and you seem to understand me.

Therapist: Are you sure this is okay with the both of you? I can always give you a referral.

Mateo: It's fine with me. I don't need any more help. I have made my decision and I feel fine with it. But for the sake of our kids, I would like her to be a little less hostile.

Mariana: I'm so confused. How can you do this to me and the kids?

Mateo: I have been warning you this day would come.

Mariana: Doctor, I do not want to start over with anyone and besides, you know the both of us. I want to stay here.

Therapist: Okay. If you both agree, I will do this. But you do realize that this will take me out of the running as your couples therapist if something changes.

Mateo: Nothing will change. Just help her.

Post-divorce, I refuse to see one of the partners with a new mate, unless the case has come to me years later with one caveat: I will never do so if the new mate was previously engaged in an affair with my former client. I prefer to remain loyal to the original couple and wish to avoid any future control struggles that could arise with the scorned ex-partner. It might also save me from mistakenly breaching a confidence that was shared in the original couple's conjoint sessions. This has cost me a few clients over the years, but I still think it is a prudent stance to take.

Couples Who Resist Terminating

Running counter to the couple that will terminate prematurely is the couple who do little to no work in treatment yet have the resources and tenacity to show up every week without fail. Prochaska and Prochaska (2008) termed this "delayed termination" or "when therapy continues even though additional benefits from therapy do not continue" (p. 151). Clinicians that set concrete treatment goals such as cognitive behavioral therapists (Jacobson, 2014; Strong, 2020) are less likely to let this dynamic go on indefinitely. In the MCT approach, however, the behavior is usually interpreted as a shared conflict about control that merits treatment no matter how long it takes. After interpreting the control conflict, it is then correlated with the couple's chief complaint, to similar struggles in other contexts, and to each partner's family of origin. Consider the following example of Jon—who presented having a long-term affair—and his wife, Kristen, who finally exposed it:

Therapist: Neither of you seem to be working awfully hard on understanding why the affair took place. And it was a long one: about three years. You come religiously but do nothing. I suspect this is a pattern. Kristen, you told me you suspected Jon was having an affair, but you never really followed up on your suspicions. And Jon, you have never sought help.

Kristen: What pattern?

Therapist: Do you know what I mean Jon?

Jon: That we don't fix our problems?

Therapist: Yes, and I think you're doing the same in treatment. Neither of you seem to have a need to get to the bottom of things here. Some therapists might praise you both for your dedication to treatment, but all you do is show up every week. I don't want to be critical. I know you both came from homes in which nothing ever improved. Your parents seemed paralyzed to deal with family problems and you both were witness to this paralysis. But now I believe this is a pattern. I believe that you are both replicating a certain resistance to fixing your problems, just as you did with the affair. But this goes even beyond the affair. Each of you have expressed problems with your careers and your children, yet you do little to address these issues. Everything is out-of-control.

Sometimes interpreting and broadening the conflict and connecting it to each partner's family of origin does not free a couple to either work in treatment or to end it. In this situation I may interpret the resistance as a control struggle with the treatment process itself and continue to do so until the couple tires or decides what to do. In some cases, an interpretation may be slightly adjusted and can make all the difference in the couple's reaction. The following is an example of Ruth and Phil, a married couple referred by a colleague after a frustrating two years of treatment. At this point the couple were in treatment with me for approximately two more years. Notice that I accepted a reinterpretation from Ruth, yet remained focused on the couple's control struggle with the treatment process:

Ruth: More than once you have told me that we're not progressing in treatment. But we have the time and the money so we would like to keep coming. Maybe something will happen at some point.

Therapist: Maybe, but it's not just about coming here, it's about doing the work.

Ruth: Well, I think our marriage is a mess and that we're powerless to do anything about it. We hope you can.

Therapist: Powerless is not the word I would use to describe you and Phil. In fact, I see you both as powerful in your reluctance to take on your marital issues.

Phil: I can't relate to the word power. I just don't feel that way.

Therapist: A lot of people think it is a negative term, but power can be used for good as well as evil.

Ruth: But not in the way you are applying it to us. I see it as negative.

Therapist: Well, maybe that is not the right word. Perhaps I see you both as "strong" people who can take on your issues if you choose to. It is your collective strength that I find so formidable.

Ruth: I can relate to that better. So, you don't think we're using our strength for our own benefit?

Therapist: Something like that. I think you are using it to try and defeat those therapists who care about you, or to defeat treatment itself.

Many therapists cannot tolerate this type of gridlock, and I seem to get many referrals from colleagues who quit on a couple like Ruth and Phil. But it is important to persevere, and to analyze the control dynamics of the relationship rather than to give up. Such resistance in conflict therapy is to be expected—even predicted. Given that each partner has internalized two opposing sides, formidable gridlock is quite normal.

The Impact of Premature Termination and Therapeutic Failure on the Couples Therapist

Therapists often blame themselves for a couple's failure to move or improve, but there is also a tendency to blame themselves if a couple prematurely drops out of treatment. Many feel a sense of failure, demoralization, or rejection (Swift & Greenberg, 2015). Others may experience sadness, confusion, disappointment, shame (Piselli et al., 2011), or loss (Patterson et al., 2018).

Self-blame cannot always be attributed to a therapist's neurotic guilt. Some therapists are burned out from work-related stressors and cannot give all couples the attention they need (Horton, 2020); other therapists are clearly overmatched in some cases and should not have experimented with a couple by taking on something that they cannot treat competently (DeAngelis, 2018). Unfortunately, this is all too common in the complex field of psychotherapy. Consider the family therapist with little to no training in couples work taking on couples, or a couples therapist with little to no sex therapy training treating couples with sexual disorders. Knowing your professional limitations is important because it is impossible to know everything.

Most therapists, however, are well-trained—some exquisitely so—and try and do the best job they can. Yet many express remorse, and even self-flagellate when they have lost a case even if they had little control and the odds were against them. Why would they take this so hard? Why would they be so upset if a couple decides to terminate prematurely or if a couple decides to divorce? With reference to psychoanalysts, Jung (1946/1966) used the term "wounded healers." He believed that analysts are compelled to enter the field because they themselves are flawed in some way. He wrote:

> We could say, without too much exaggeration, that a good half of every treatment that probes at all deeply consists in the doctor's examining himself, for only what he can put right in himself can he hope to put right in the patient. It is no loss, either, if he feels that the patient is hitting him, or even scoring off him: it is his own hurt that gives the measure of his power to heal. This, and nothing else, is the meaning of the Greek myth of the wounded physician.
>
> (p. 238)

Straussner et al. (2018) wrote "that helping professionals are disproportionately affected by behavioral health problems" (p. 1). Focusing on licensed social workers, the authors found that 40.2% of the respondents of a large-scale survey reported mental health problems before becoming social workers and 51.8% during their careers. Zerubavel and Wright (2012) created a framework for practicing psychologists, distinguishing between wounded healers who can use their issues to help clients and those practitioners whose emotional problems negatively impact their psychotherapy practice. But perhaps psychiatrist Tena Moyer (2021) made the point in the bluntest of terms: "I am a psychiatrist because, when I was growing up, my mother was crazy. It really is that simple" (p. 24).

Many therapists were parentified in their respective families of origin (Boszormenyi-Nagy & Spark, 1973). In earlier studies, Sessions (1986) found that graduate psychology students scored higher on parentification measures than graduate engineering students. Lackie (1983) reported that two-thirds of the social workers he studied had histories of caretaking. Prior to professional training, these caregivers may have mediated their parents' squabbles when growing up; played the role of the caretaking parent to their siblings; or were called upon to make up for their parents' general incompetence. While somewhat different, these tasks do share some common characteristics: (1) they were serious jobs and were treated as such; (2) they were age-inappropriate at the time; (3) they were impossible to do perfectly; (4) there was little reward for doing these jobs; and (5) if not completed to expectation it was considered by other family members to be a punishable offense. Any one of these experiences can produce fine administrators and decision makers, sensitive and empathic individuals, and of course, people intuitive beyond their years—the very makings of a therapist. But they can also lead to an overworked clinician with an overdeveloped sense of responsibility which can flare when they disappoint clients.

Being aware of and controlling this vulnerability is easier said than done—because ultimately it may entail the therapist realizing that his/her parents perhaps were not assigned enough responsibility for their pathology. Nevertheless, the couple's therapist must take appropriate responsibility for the treatment and leave the rest to the couple. They must accept that they only have so much control over the couple and the therapeutic process, or they will end up out-of-control. For years I have told my young supervisees that the sooner they realize how little control they have over a couple, the better the couples therapist they will be.

Relapse Prevention

Relapse Prevention (RE), first credited to Marlatt and George (1984), is a cognitive-behavioral concept which focuses on the maintenance of habit change. While most often applied to controlling various addictions (Hendershot et al., 2011), McCarthy (2001) recommends this approach with couples who suffer from sexual disorders. Likewise, in MCT I recommend certain strategies to help couples to stay in control of their conflict and to keep symptoms, sexual and nonsexual, at a minimum. I especially remind the couple of the following at the time of termination:

- *Expect flareups*: Because there is no cure for an unbalanced conflict following formal treatment, the couple should expect flareups. They should not be as intense and frequent as they were prior to treatment, but they will occur from time to time. The couple must remember that the goal is not to completely eradicate this conflict, only their symptoms. And this should occur if their conflict is rebalanced.
- *Shared conflict*: Because both partners have the same conflict, they should refrain from blaming each other for additional flareups.
- *Think conflict*: If a flareup occurs, do not escalate it by focusing exclusively on content. Rather, immediately consider the process and think conflict.
- *Booster sessions*: While a gradual termination process should give the therapist a chance to judge how a couple will do on their own, a booster session or two may be recommended in a few months. This is especially important if the therapist has some reservations about the couple's control issues. The couple should welcome this checkup.
- *Tune-ups*: If there is a need to return to treatment because new symptoms have appeared, schedule a tune-up. More than likely the conflict has resurfaced and in a new context but can be easily rebalanced. Do not be embarrassed to return for a tune-up.
- *Stay positive*: Having had the tenacity and perseverance to rebalance a conflict and alleviate symptoms related to a control struggle in treatment, it is usually easier to get it quickly back under control thereafter. Be confident and hopeful. According to Swift and Greenberg (2015), hope is what motivates clients to continue their therapeutic journey.

References

Bartle-Haring, S., Glebova, T., Gangamma, R., Grafsky, E., & Delaney, R. (2012). Alliance and termination status in couple therapy: A comparison of methods for assessing discrepancies. *Psychotherapy Research, 22,* 502–514. https://doi.org/10.1080/10503307.2012.676985

Betchen, S., & Davidson, H. (2018). *Master conflict therapy: A new model for practicing couples and sex therapy.* Routledge.

Björk, T., Bjorck, C., Clinton, D., Sohlberg, D., & Norring, C. (2009). What happened to the ones who dropped out? Outcome in eating disorder clients who complete or prematurely terminate treatment. *European Eating Disorder Review, 17,* 109–119. https://doi.org/10.1002/erv.911

Boszormenyi-Nagy, I., & Spark, G. (1973). *Invisible loyalties.* Harper & Row.

Bowen, M. (1978). *Family therapy in clinical practice.* Aronson.

Cummings, N. (2008). Interruption replaces termination in focused, intermittent psychotherapy throughout the life cycle. In W.T. O'Donohue & M.A. Cucciare (Eds.), *Terminating psychotherapy* (pp. 99–119). Routledge.

DeAngelis, T. (2018, May). What should you do if a case is outside your skill set? *Monitor on Psychology, 49*(5). www.apa.org/monitor/2018/05/ce-corner

Doss, B.D., Hsueh, A.C., & Carhart, K. (2011). Premature termination in couple therapy with veterans: Veterans: Definitions and prediction of long-term outcomes. *Journal of Family Psychology, 25,* 770–774. https://doi.org/10.1037/a0025239

Greenan, D. (2010). Therapy with a gay male couple: An unlikely multisystemic integration. In A. Gurman (Ed.), *Clinical casebook of couple therapy* (5th ed., pp. 90–111). Guilford Press.

Heitler, S. (2013, October 28). Individual therapy for married people: A huge mistake? *Psychology Today.* www.psychologytoday.com/us/blog/resolution-not-conflict/201310/individual-therapy-married-people-huge-mistake

Hendershot, C.S., Witkiewitz, K., George, W.H., & Marlatt, G.A. (2011). Relapse prevention for addictive behaviors. *Substance Abuse Treatment Prevalence Policy, 6,* 6–17. https://doi.org/10.1186/1747-597X-6-17

Horton, A.P. (2020, March 6). *How burnout affects mental health workers.* BBC Worklife. www.bbc.com/worklife/article/20200305-how-burnout-affects-mental-health-workers

Jacobson, S. (2014, April 15). *Cognitive behavioral therapy techniques demystified.* Harley Therapy. www.regain.us/advice/therapist/how-do-couples-therapists-use-cognitive-behavioral-therapy/.

Jung, C.G. (1946/1966). The practice of psychotherapy: Essays on the psychology of the transference and other subjects. Fundamental questions of psychotherapy. In H. Read, M. Fordham, G. Adler, & W. McGuire (Eds.), R.F.C. Hull (Trans.), *The collected works of C.G. Jung* (2nd ed.) (Vol. 16, pp. 163–240). Princeton University Press.

Jurek, J., Janusz, B., Chwal, M., & de Barbaro, B. (2014). Premature termination in couple therapy as part of therapeutic process: Cross case analysis. *Archives of Psychiatry and Psychotherapy, 16,* 51–59. https://doi.org/10.12740/APP/26962

Lackie, B. (1983). The families of origin of social workers. *Clinical Social Work Journal, 11,* 309–322. https://doi.org/10.1007/BF00755898

Marlatt, G.A., & George, W.H. (1984). Relapse prevention: Introduction and overview of the model. *British Journal of Addiction, 79,* 261–273. https://doi.org/10.1111/j.1360-0443.1984.tb00274.x

McCarthy, B. (2001). Relapse prevention strategies and techniques with erectile disorder. *Journal or Sex & Marital Therapy, 27*, 1–8. https://doi.org/10.180/00926230152035804

Morrill, M., & Córdova, J. (2010). Building intimacy bridges: From the marriage checkup to integrative behavioral couple therapy. In A. Gurman (Ed.)., *Clinical casebook for couple therapy* (pp. 331–354). Guilford.

Moyer, T. (2021, September/October). The art of repairing broken things. *Psychology Today*, 22–25.

Patterson, J., Williams, L., Edwards, T.M., Chamow, L., & Grauf-Grounds, C. (2018). *Essential skills in family therapy: From the first interview to termination*. Guilford.

Piselli, A., Halgin, R.P., & MacEwan, G.H. (2011). What went wrong? Therapists' reflections on their role in premature termination. *Psychotherapy Research, 21*, 400–415. https://doi.org/10.1080/10503307.2011.573819

Prochaska, J., & Prochaska, J. (2008). Termination at each stage of change. In W.T. O'Donohue & M.A. Cucciare (Eds.), *Terminating psychotherapy* (pp. 147–162). Routledge.

Sessions, M.W. (1986). *Influence of parentification on professional role choice and interpersonal style* [Doctoral dissertation, Georgia State University]. Dissertation Abstracts International, 47, 5066. (University Microfilms No. 87–06815).

Siegel, J. (2010). A good-enough therapy: An object relations approach. In A. Gurman (Ed.), *Clinical casebook of couple therapy* (5th ed., pp. 134–152). Guilford.

Straussner, S.L.A., Senreich, E., & Steen, J. (2018). Wounded healers: A multistate study of licensed social workers' behavioral problems. *Social Work, 63*, 125–133. https://doi.org/10.1093/sw/swy012

Strong, E. (2020, August 5). *How do couples therapists use cognitive behavioral therapy?* www.regain.us/advice/therapist/how-do-couples-therapists-use-cognitive-behavioral-therapy/

Swift, J., & Greenberg, R. (2012). Premature discontinuation in adult psychotherapy: A meta-analysis. *Journal of Consulting and Clinical Psychology, 80*, 547–559. https://doi.org/10/1037/a0028226

Swift, J., & Greenberg, R. (2015). *Premature termination in psychotherapy: Strategies for engaging clients and improving outcomes*. American Psychological Association.

Swift, J., Spencer, J., & Goode, J. (2018). Improving psychotherapy effectiveness by addressing the problem of premature termination: Introduction to a special section. *Psychotherapy Research, 28*, 669–671. https://doi.org/10.1080/10503307.2018.1439192

Tartakovsky, M. (2016, Mat 17). *Therapists spill: How to end therapy*. PsychCentral. https://psychcentral.com/lib/therapists-spill-how-to-end-therapy#1

Wachtel, E. (2017). *The heart of couple therapy: Knowing what to do and when to do it*. Guilford.

Zerubavel, N., & Wright, M.O. (2012). The dilemma of the wounded healer. *Psychotherapy, 49*, 482–491. https://doi.org/10.1037/a0027824

Epilogue

Several years ago, I mentioned to a colleague that one day I would write "the" book on couples therapy—a book that would be in every graduate-school class-room on the subject. Without hesitation she said: "There is no such thing. Therapists follow different models and basically have their own way of practicing. This is not urology, where most physicians follow a similar protocol. I am sure you will attract some followers, but to think in grandiose terms is simply unrealistic." Accepting my colleague's rational explanation, and feeling less grandiose as a result, I immediately began to ponder what "would" be useful to all those practicing couples therapy. What concept would resonate with most?

I eventually, albeit humbly, decided to choose a specific dynamic that every couples therapist must face on a regular basis; and one that, despite its frequency, had not been the subject of a professional book: the infamous *pursuer-distancer* dynamic originally conceived of by Bowen (1978) and Fogarty (1979) and credited in the literature as the cause of more divorces than any other dynamic (Hetherington & Kelly, 2003). Fortunately, my idea proved to be as popular as I thought, and the book is still in print (Betchen, 2005). I expanded the work on the dynamic both theoretically and clinically much to the appreciation of Thomas Fogarty, who sent me a heartfelt letter of appreciation for my work to which I was honored.

Even as I worked diligently over the next few years to develop the MCT model (Betchen, 2010), I kept my newfound approach in mind, focusing on which specific conflict seemed to be the most common one presented by couples in treatment. That is, which conflict showed itself as often as the pursuer-distancer dynamic, and likewise, was given no more than scant attention in the professional literature. The result: *control versus out-of-control*.

In over 40 years of treating couples, with an average of 30–40 per week, I determined that the concept of control was vital in understanding how a couple's symptoms are produced and maintained. And in studying this concept, I was genuinely surprised that not a single professional book on the subject is available to guide couples therapists in this endeavor. Many commercial or popular books (Evans, 2002; Parrott, 2000; Rose, 2013; Simon, 1996; Viorst, 1998) are, but none written specifically for couples therapists. Because this omission met the new criteria I set for my scholarly and professional work, I proceeded to spend a lot of time thinking and writing about the concept of control.

One of the most important tenets of control that I touched on in "Chapter 1. Control and Conflict," seems to run counter to the way many view the concept: that people who try too hard to maintain control in their relationships and in their lives often lose control. Remember the example of the controlling husband who set strict limits on how much his wife could spend until she rebelled and went on a spending spree. Even when I expanded the relational context into sexual dynamics, I found this paradox to remain valid. Consider the woman I treated who controlled the sex in her relationship by exerting many rules and regulations about sexual frequency, style, and substance. In response, her once passive husband left her for a more sexually open neighbor.

Why would a reasonably intelligent individual exert control in a situation where the opposite would be merited? When in trouble, controlling people tend to try and cure their problem by treating it with whatever caused the problem to begin with. These people see "the poison as the cure." It is as if they know only one way to live; one way to solve life's problems. Even if you specifically tell this person what bothers you about them, rather than change, they intensify the behavior. It may seem illogical to most, but these individuals may wholeheartedly believe that this action will solve the problem, even though it almost always makes it worse. Healthier or less controlling individuals may, on a subconscious level, be aware that their tactic will fail, but nevertheless, they are compelled to do what it is they "think" they do best. They use the one tool they have in their toolbox.

I have found the following metaphor from the automotive world useful to consider in treating a couple that is stuck in control struggle: controlling people often seem to be missing a second gear; they only have a first and third gear. In first gear, they are just starting and are not yet locked into position. In this gear they can be open to suggestion because they are aware of how little they know. But soon enough they choose their destination and desired speed, and lock into third gear, skipping over the more moderate position of second gear. But without second gear, these people are more rigid and less likely to compromise. As a result, they are left particularly vulnerable to their internal conflict and may sabotage whatever control they did have. In this sense, they insist on driving too fast for their own good and refuse to listen to anyone who tries to slow them down.

I believe that considering the concept of control from a conflict perspective adds an originality to the way couples therapists can think about control struggles in relationships. The fact that this approach also allows for the integration of sex therapy makes it an even more useful approach to treating a diverse group of couples (Betchen & Davidson, 2018). I also believe that this perspective can apply to the clinical supervision process. For example, less experienced supervisees, unless oppositional by nature, tend to take in their supervisor's suggestions or directives. But older, more experienced supervisees—settled into previous training habits—may put up a bit more resistance, thus mirroring the therapeutic dynamic between the supervisor and an actual couple (Betchen, 1995). The less differentiated both parties are, the more likely this is to happen (Bowen,

1978). Just as with client-couples, the more supervisor and supervisee match up in terms of style and approach, the less room there will be for a control struggle.

It is not unusual, however, for a supervisee trained in a behavioral approach to seek out a more psychodynamic model only to have some degree of difficulty grasping or even accepting it. When faced with formidable resistance in supervision, the supervisor can point out that the two of them may be locked into a control struggle. This might even apply to a disagreement about general therapeutic interventions which may call for the supervisor to take a more extreme approach. For example, a supervisee refused to refer his client for alcohol treatment after I had strongly recommended that he do so. The client was experiencing blackouts and I felt the situation was dangerous to all parties. However, the supervisee, claiming to have some experience with substance treatment, refused to comply, forcing me to order him to make the referral. When he continued to resist, I offered that he and I were engaged in a control struggle and if he did not pull back, I would have to take clinical control from him and suspend supervision. He finally acquiesced and we later discovered a pattern of his taking control and losing it that was eventually helpful to the supervision process.

A second example is that of a female supervisee who refused to collect her fees from a couple she felt sorry for because of their precarious financial situation. Because we were in a clinic at the time, and the clinic depended on client fees to function, this needed to be dealt with as soon as possible. Nevertheless, the supervisee refused to charge this couple until she was threatened to be fired from the clinic. I pointed out to her that by fighting so hard to maintain control, as she saw fit, she could have lost her job and with it, control over her career.

Control is a universal concept that it is important in almost every part of our lives. I have, on occasion, been asked by clients to apply it to sports. A client who was focused on lowering his golf score would often try so hard that he tightened up before important shots and he would inevitably misplay them. He admitted to me that the more he tried to control his game the worse he seemed to play. Others may want control over the outcome so badly that they cheat and in turn, end up disgraced.

In the world of business, those managers who drive their underlings to strive for perfection often burn them out and in turn, experience less productivity. Those that demand so much control may be difficult to talk to. Many are simply closed to new ideas and as a result, may thwart employee creativity and self-worth. A friend in the business world had worked at a company for almost 20 years as a salesman but desperately wanted to move into management. Although he had done very well in sales, his bosses refused to promote him despite his complaining. One day we met at a restaurant and he threw a stack of papers on the table and asked me to interpret them. The papers turned out to be the results of several psychological tests that the company often gave to prospective high-level managers. Apparently, my friend's boss got tired of his whining and had the human resource department test him. The results strongly indicated the very thing that I had been telling my friend for years: "When his mouth opens, your ears close." Simply put, these tests showed my friend to be rigid, stubborn, and controlling, and that he would make a terrible manager.

Control also operates on a macro level, which has perhaps never been more evident than today. Groups have formed and people have chosen sides in a way that harkens back to civil war times. The term "identity politics" is used by many to explain why it is that people choose a side even if it does not make sense to do so in a certain context. For example, my friends wonder why it is that our two major political parties not only are warring with each other, but internally as well. They wonder why both parties seemed to politicize a bi-partisan virus. The answer is control. You cannot run the country until your party has won office. The real control starts there.

In sum, my objective in writing this book was not to sway couples therapists to practice my specific model of treatment. It was to offer *one* perspective on the concept of control. I have found it to be pervasive in the lives of couples; play a part in partner choice; transcendent of race, culture, and sexual orientation; complex and paradoxical; responsible for a couple's gridlock and a wide variety of symptoms; and highly responsive to treatment. At the very least, if I have been able to help some therapists to pay more attention to the concept in the treatment process, this will have been worth the effort.

References

Betchen, S. (1995). An integrative, intersystemic approach to supervision of couple therapy. *American Journal of Family Therapy*, *23*, 48–58. https://doi.org/10.1080/01926189508251335

Betchen, S. (2005). *Intrusive partners-elusive mates: The pursuer distancer dynamic in couples therapy*. Routledge.

Betchen, S. (2010). *Magnetic partners: Discover how the hidden conflict that once attracted you to each other is now driving you apart*. Free Press.

Betchen, S., & Davidson, H. (2018). *Master conflict therapy: A new model for practicing couples and sex therapy*. Routledge.

Bowen, M. (1978). *Family therapy in clinical practice*. Aronson.

Evans, P. (2002). *Controlling people: How to recognize, understand, and deal with people who try to control you*. Adams Media.

Fogarty, T. (1979). The distance and the pursuer. *The Family*, *7*, 11–16.

Hetherington, E.M., & Kelly, J. (2003). *For better or for worse: Divorce reconsidered*. Norton & Company.

Parrott, L. (2000). *The control freak*. Tyndale House Publishers, Inc.

Rose, M. (2013). *Power & control in relationships*. Vase Publishing.

Simon, G. (1996). *In sheep's clothing: Understanding and dealing with manipulative people*. A.J. Christopher & Company.

Viorst, J. (1998). *Imperfect control*. Simon & Schuster.

Index

Page numbers in *italics* indicate figures.

double binds 147–149
drug disorders 50–51
DSM-5 *see Diagnostic and Statistical Manual of Mental Disorders* (DSM-5)

Emotionally Focused Therapy (EFS) 31, 82
emotional manipulation 39–40
enabling 12, 41–43
erectile dysfunction (ED) 63, 90–91
external conflict 6–7, 72
extramarital affairs 33–35, 66
eye rolling 48

Fairbairn, W.R.D. 8, 29
family of origin: connecting conflict to 164; contradictory messages and 17–23; control struggles and 5–6, 17–23; mate preference and 31; roles in 65
feigning deafness 48
female orgasmic disorder 92, 132–134
Ferrari, J. 48
fetishes 65
financial control: conflict and 12; parents who contradict each other 22–23; techniques of 43–45; women victims of 43–44
Fisher, H. 28
flirtatious behavior 45
Fogarty, T. 170
Ford, A. 14
Fox, J. 149
Freud, S. 8, 28, 77
Frisby, B.N. 45

gambling addiction 50–51
Gander, K. 14
Ganesh and Indira (staying married) case: arranged marriage and 111–112, 116–117; broadening context of conflict 115–116; control struggles and 111–113; examining families of origin 116–117; exposing conflict with control 114–115; exposing control struggle 113–114; genogram *112*; increasing differentiation 117–118; integrating internal conflict 117–118
gender equality 13–14
Genito-Pelvic/Pain Penetration Disorder (GPPPD) 66–67, 92
genograms: control struggle assessment 62–66; Deshawn and Shanice (domestic chores/division of labor) case *105*; Ganesh and Indira (staying married) case *112*; Hank and Diane (nonsexual control

struggle) case *69*, 71–72; Jordan and Cheryl (sexual control struggle) case *73*, 75–76; Ray and Joan (procrastination) case *94*; Robert and Jonathan (MHSDD) case *119*; Sandy and Joel (delayed ejaculation) case *127, 133*
George, W.H. 167
Gottman, J. 39
Gray, D. 58
Greenberg, R. 167

Hank and Diane (nonsexual control struggle) case: chief complaint 68–69, *69*; content versus process 72; control versus out-of-control conflict and 71–72; financial control conflict 69, *69*, 70–72; first session 69–71; genogram *69*, 71–72; initial contact 68–69
Harris, S. 60
Hartog, H. 13
Hazan, C. 30
Heffernan, M. 29
Holmes, B. 30
Horney, K. 8
Horowitz, L.M. 30
Howard, K. 14

Imperfect Control (Viorst) 12
in-home exercises 83, 92
integrative therapy 127
internal conflict: abusive relationships and 41; awareness of 7–8; control and 7–9, 18, 23; external symptoms and 8; master conflicts and 35; mate preference and 34–35; metamessages and 17; psychological symptoms and 8–9; subpersonalities and 8–9; unbalanced 37; *see also* Master Conflict Therapy (MCT)
Internal Family Systems (IFS) 8–9, 82
interpersonal differentiation 31
intrapsychic differentiation 31
intuition 149

Jantz, G. 45
Johnson, K. 30
Johnson, S. 31
Johnson, V. 83
joining 146–147
Jordan and Cheryl (sexual control struggle) case: chief complaint 72, *73*; content versus process 76; control versus out-of-control conflict and 76; first session 72–75; genogram *73*, 75–76; initial

contact 72; passive-aggressive behavior
74–75; sexual assessment 73–76
Jung, C.G. 28, 166
Jurek, J. 162

Kaplan, H.S. 63, 83, 93
Karson, M. 82
Klein, M. 29
Klingsieck, K. 48
Kohut, H. 146
Koskimki, J. 90
Kupferman, E. 42

Lackie, B. 166
Lancer, D. 49
Lee, C. 64, 113
Linn, A. 151
low sexual desire 82, 120–121

male hypoactive sexual desire disorder
(MHSDD) 90, 118, 120, 126
marital rape 46
Marlatt, G.A. 167
Martin, S. 42
masculinity 39, 109, 111
master conflicts: acceptance of 157;
balanced 10, *10*; comfortable balance
11; control versus out-of-control 11–13,
35, 71–72, 76–77; internal duality and
9, 19, 35; partner unbalancing of 9–10;
unbalanced *11*
Master Conflict Therapy (MCT): control
struggles and 82, 91; control versus
out-of-control conflict and 170; couple
exercises 91–92; criteria for termination
of treatment 157–159; delayed ejaculation
treatment 127; insight-focused treatment
in 91–92; integrating internal conflict
101; mate preference and 32–35;
premature termination of treatment 162;
premise of 9; relapse prevention and 167;
resistance to termination of treatment
164; sex therapy exercises 133; similarity
in couples 33; therapeutic objectives 91;
therapist conflict with control 155
Masters, W. 83
masturbation 65, 92
mate preference: attachment theory and
30–31; biological factors in 28; control
struggles and 27; family of origin and
31; internal conflict and 34–35; MCT
and 32–35; Object Relations therapy and
29–30; psychoanalytic theory and 28–29;

sexual selection and 27–28; systems
therapy and 31; unconscious process of
27–35
McCabe, M.P. 92
McCarthy, B. 167
McFarlane, A.C. 24
MCT *see* Master Conflict Therapy (MCT)
meditation 91
metamessages 17
#MeToo movement 14
MHSDD *see* male hypoactive sexual desire
disorder (MHSDD)
mindfulness techniques 91
Mintz, L. 92
"mixed-agenda" couples 60
Moyer, T. 166
multicultural population 113
multigenerational transmission process 6, 157

Nagoski, E. 92
National Center for Drug Abuse Statistics
(NCDAS) 50
New Male Sexuality, The (Zilbergeld) 83
Nimbi, F.M. 120
non-threatening intervention 82

Object Relations Therapy 8, 29–30
obsessive compulsive disorder (OCD) 5
orgasm: female orgasmic disorder 92,
132–134; inhibited 72–73, *73*, 74, 76

paraphilias 65
parentification: Contextual Therapy and
82; control struggles and 19, 21, 64–65,
82, 110; impact on relationships 82;
responsibilities and 19, 64–65, 108;
therapists and 166
Park, D. 113
Parrot, L. 49
passive-aggressive behavior 49–50
Perrett, D. 29
physical abuse 38, 40–41; *see also* domestic
violence
physical attraction 28, 65
Pikiewicz, K. 41
porn 51, 57, 65
post-conflict trauma 25
post-traumatic stress disorder (PTSD) 23–24
pre-conflict trauma 24–25
preliminary hypothesis 82–83
premature ejaculation (PE) 92, 161
premature termination 159–162, 165–167
preoccupied attachment 30

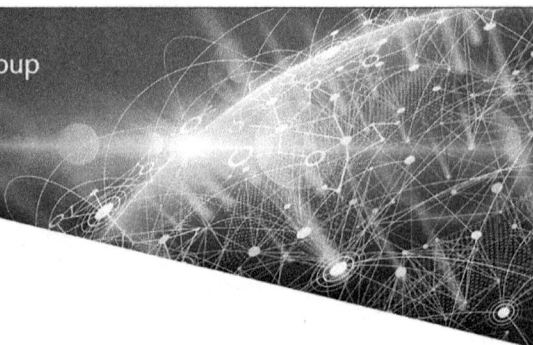

For Product Safety Concerns and Information please contact our EU
representative GPSR@taylorandfrancis.com
Taylor & Francis Verlag GmbH, Kaufingerstraße 24, 80331 München, Germany